ACHIEVING DISTINCTION IN NURSING EDUCATION

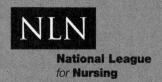

National League
for **Nursing**

ACHIEVING DISTINCTION IN NURSING EDUCATION

Edited by:

Marsha Howell Adams, PhD, RN, CNE, FAAN, ANEF

Theresa M. Valiga, EdD, RN, CNE, FAAN, ANEF

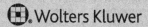

. Wolters Kluwer

Philadelphia · Baltimore · New York · London
Buenos Aires · Hong Kong · Sydney · Tokyo

Vice President, Nursing Segment: Julie K. Stegman
Manager, Nursing Education and Practice Content: Jamie Blum
Senior Development Editor: Meredith L. Brittain
Marketing Manager: Greta H. Swanson
Editorial Assistant: Molly Kennedy
Manager, Graphic Arts and Design: Steve Druding
Senior Production Project Manager: Sadie Buckallew
Manufacturing Coordinator: Margie Orzech
Prepress Vendor: S4Carlisle Publishing Services

Adams, M. H., & Valiga, T. M. (2022). *Achieving distinction in nursing education.* National League for Nursing.

9 8 7 6 5 4 3 2 1

Printed in the United States of America

Library of Congress Cataloging-in-Publication Data

ISBN-13: 978-1-9751-8500-8
ISBN-10: 1-9751-8500-5
Library of Congress Control Number: 2021910985

Cataloging-in-Publication data available on request from the Publisher.

DRC0821

This book is dedicated to nursing faculty, staff, and students who dedicate themselves every day to striving for excellence and distinction within themselves and through their nursing programs. It is also dedicated to all future nurse educators who are open to thinking out of the box to achieve excellence and who want to make every effort to demonstrate excellence professionally. Finally, I want to dedicate this book to my husband of 44 years, Phil, for always loving and supporting me in my many endeavors. To my three sons — Abe, Tom, and Jon — who are always in my corner, making me smile and appreciate life, and who gave me seven beautiful grandchildren. I continue to be blessed having all these individuals in my life.

MA

This book is dedicated to the many individuals who have supported, challenged, and guided me throughout a long and successful career as a nurse educator. The hundreds of students I've taught over the years have inspired me with their spirit of inquiry, desire to learn, and passion for nursing. The many faculty colleagues with whom I have had the privilege of working have helped me clarify my thinking and validated the importance of collaborative efforts as, together, we presented at professional conferences, published, conducted research, and created innovative curricula and learning experiences. The diverse colleagues with whom I have worked in various professional associations illustrate the many ways in which we are similar, as well as the ways in which differences can be "tapped" to realize a vision. And finally, I want to dedicate this book to my family. Although my parents are no longer with us, they always encouraged me to take risks, strive to do my very best, and look for the good in others. My sister, Diane, a nurse herself, has been a role model nurse and leader, and I will always be grateful for her. And I cannot express how truly grateful I am to my husband, Bob, who has consistently supported and encouraged me for more than 50 years, from those early days in graduate school through many years of a "commuter marriage," where I worked in one state and our permanent home was in another, and into retirement; he truly is a treasure.

TV

Achieving Distinction in Nursing Education: Reflections from the National League for Nursing President and CEO

Interestingly, "distinction" is a synonym for "excellence," so the book's title could read *Achieving Excellence in Nursing Education*. The journey for excellence and distinction began long before my time of service at the National League for Nursing (NLN). Founded in 1893 as the first nursing organization in the United States, NLN acquired the honor of distinguishing itself as the birth mother of all U.S. nursing organizations. NLN's initial name was the American Society of Superintendents of Training Schools for Nurses, and nursing education has remained the primary focus and raison d'etre of the NLN's existence over its lifetime.

NLN's North Star, or mission, is to promote excellence in nursing education to build a strong and diverse nursing workforce to advance the health of the nation and the global community. There is a clear recognition in the statement that although education is critical, it cannot stand alone but must be connected by bridges of practice to the health of the diverse people nurses serve throughout the world. In other words, although the NLN was born in the United States, it belongs to the global community and acknowledges that America's health is only as good as the health of its international "others." The COVID-19 worldwide pandemic has demonstrated this as perhaps no other testimonial could.

A mission statement, however, is not enough to qualify for the honor of distinction. Distinction requires implementation. The NLN implements its mission guided by four dynamic and integrated core values that permeate the organization and are reflected in its work, its members and staff, and even the structure of its building. When the NLN moved from New York City to Washington, DC, it required architectural changes to its new office space. There was an intentional design decision to include the four distinctive core values in the actual building itself. Consequently, surrounding the boardroom at the NLN are the core values etched in glass to remind those who work daily of the commitment required and to provide those who visit with a clear statement of the platform on which the NLN is built. These four core values are as follows:

▸ **Caring** is promoting health, healing, and hope in response to the human condition. This culture of caring, a fundamental part of the nursing profession, characterizes the NLN's concern and consideration for the whole person, commitment to the common good, and outreach to those who are vulnerable. The goal is for all organizational activities to be managed in a participative and person-centered way, demonstrating an ability to understand and appreciate the needs of others.

> **Integrity** is respecting the dignity and moral wholeness of every person without conditions or limitation. This culture is evident when organizational principles of open communication, ethical decision-making, and humility are encouraged, expected, and demonstrated consistently. NLN strives to see itself from the perspective of others in a larger community, resulting in a commitment to truth telling and a deliberate effort to keep the business of doing the right thing at the front of the NLN agenda.

> **Diversity with Inclusion** is affirming the uniqueness of and differences among persons, ideas, values, and ethnicities. This represents a mark of distinction as the NLN continually assesses its diversity with inclusion for every aspect of the organization, from its members and programs to its staff and leadership. Knowing that differences affect innovation, new dialogues can serve to challenge old systems that have built-in structures of racism and other "isms" and co-create new structures. By acknowledging the legitimacy and necessity of us all, there can be movement beyond mere tolerance to valued engagement and celebration of the richness that differences bring forth.

> **Excellence** is co-creating and implementing transformative strategies with daring ingenuity, a value that integrates the other three values. There is no excellence without caring, integrity, and diversity with inclusion. Although co-creation is essential, the requirement for the implementation of transformative strategies is equally necessary. Excellence extends beyond change to the amplification of the outcome, demanding more than expected and requiring leaps into unknown territory.

The NLN's mission and its commitment to these values press the mark of distinction onto the NLN's persona. Distinguishing the NLN, the *Hallmarks of Excellence in Nursing Education*© can easily be seen from any distance in time. From 1893 to 2021 and beyond, the NLN brings a culture of excellence reflecting a commitment to continuous growth, improvement, and understanding of one another. The NLN culture is where the status quo and mediocrity are not acceptable, and transformation is embraced.

Beverly Malone, PhD, RN, FAAN

About the Editors

Marsha Howell Adams, PhD, RN, CNE, FAAN, ANEF is a professor
and dean at the University of Alabama in Huntsville College of Nursing.
Dr. Adams served as the co-editor and co-author of the National League
for Nursing (NLN) publication *Achieving Excellence in Nursing Education*.
Dr. Adams has served in numerous other administrative positions over
her 39-year academic nursing career including senior associate dean
of academic programs, interim assistant dean of graduate programs,
and assistant dean of undergraduate programs while employed at the
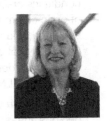
University of Alabama Capstone College of Nursing in Tuscaloosa, Alabama. Dr. Adams
received a BSN, MSN, and PhD-Nursing Education Administration from the University of
Alabama School of Nursing at Birmingham. She earned a Post-Doctoral Certificate in Rural
Case Management from the University of Alabama, Capstone College of Nursing. Dr. Adams
is a past president of the NLN (2013-2015) and the Alabama Council of Administrators of
Professional Nursing Education Programs. She is a certified nurse educator, a Fellow in the
Academy of Nursing Education, and a Fellow in the American Academy of Nursing. In 2018,
she was awarded the Alabama State Nurses Association Outstanding Nurse Administrator
Award. In 2017, she was inducted into the State of Alabama Nursing Hall of Fame. In 2018,
Dr. Adams was appointed to the National Advisory Council on Nursing Education and Practice
for a four-year term by the secretary of health and human services, Washington, DC. In 2021,
Dr. Adams was selected as on of the top 70 visionary leaders by the University of Alabama
in Birmingham School of Nursing. Dr. Adams has an extensive record of publications,
presentations, and research focusing on nursing education and health disparities of rural
women and children.

Theresa M. "Terry" Valiga, EdD, RN, CNE, FAAN, ANEF received
her bachelor's degree from Trenton State College and her master
of education and doctor of education degrees (both in Nursing
Education) from Teachers College, Columbia University. She is
professor emerita at the Duke University School of Nursing, having
served as director of their Institute for Educational Excellence and
chair of their Division of Clinical Systems and Analytics until her
retirement in August 2017. Immediately prior to her appointment at
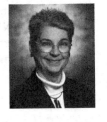
Duke, Terry served as the chief program officer at the NLN. Before that, she served on the
faculty and held administrative positions in five universities over a 26-year period: Trenton
State College, Seton Hall University, Georgetown University, Villanova University, and
Fairfield University, where she was the dean of the School of Nursing for four years. Terry
has completed research related to student learning, cognitive/intellectual development,
curriculum design, leadership development, student perspectives of excellent teachers,
and student evaluations of courses and teachers. She has received grants to support
scholarly endeavors, published extensively on a variety of leadership and education-
related topics, co-authored five books (one on leadership is now in its sixth edition),

presented papers and workshops at national and international conferences, served as a consultant to many schools of nursing inside and outside the United States, and provided leadership in several professional organizations. She has received the NLN's Outstanding Leadership in Nursing Education Award and Sigma's Elizabeth Russell Belford Founders Award for Excellence in Nursing Education, and she is a Fellow in the American Academy of Nursing and the NLN's Academy of Nursing Education.

About the Contributors

Marsha Howell Adams, PhD, RN, CNE, FAAN, ANEF is a professor and dean at the University of Alabama in Huntsville College of Nursing and served as the co-editor and co-author of the National League for Nursing (NLN) publication *Achieving Excellence in Nursing Education*. 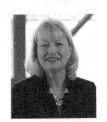 Dr. Adams has served in numerous other administrative positions over her 39-year academic nursing career including senior associate dean of academic programs, interim assistant dean of graduate programs, and assistant dean of undergraduate programs while employed at the University of Alabama Capstone College of Nursing in Tuscaloosa, Alabama. She received a BSN, MSN, and PhD-Nursing Education Administration from the University of Alabama School of Nursing at Birmingham, and she earned a Post-Doctoral Certificate in Rural Case Management from the University of Alabama, Capstone College of Nursing. Dr. Adams is a past president of the NLN (2013-2015) and the Alabama Council of Administrators of Professional Nursing Education Programs. She is a certified nurse educator, a Fellow in the Academy of Nursing Education, and a Fellow in the American Academy of Nursing. In 2017, she was inducted into the State of Alabama Nursing Hall of Fame, and in 2018, she was awarded the Alabama State Nurses Association Outstanding Nurse Administrator Award. Also, in 2018, Dr. Adams was appointed by the secretary of health and human services, Washington, DC to a four-year term on the National Advisory Council on Nursing Education and Practice. In 2021, Dr. Adams was selected as on of the top 70 visionary leaders by the University of Alabama in Birmingham School of Nursing. Dr. Adams has an extensive record of publications, presentations, and research focusing on nursing education and health disparities of rural women and children.

Janice Brewington, PhD, RN, FAAN is the chief program officer and director for the Center for Transformational Leadership at the NLN, where she developed and implemented two year-long leadership programs. 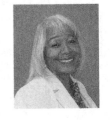 For three years prior to these responsibilities, she served the NLN as chief program officer and senior director for research and professional development. She was provost and vice chancellor for academic affairs at North Carolina Agricultural and Technical State University. While at NC A&T State University, she had a unique opportunity to be an "executive on loan" for 18 months with the Gillette Company in Boston, where she was employed as manager for university relations in talent acquisition, human resources, global shared services, North America. Her educational background includes a BSN from NC A&T State University, an MSN from Emory University, and a PhD in Health Policy and Administration from the School of Public Health, with a minor in Organizational Behavior from the School of Business, at the University of North Carolina at Chapel Hill. She also received a certificate from the Management and Leadership Institute at Harvard University and is a Fellow in the American Academy of Nursing. Dr. Brewington has provided organizational development consultation services to nonprofit businesses, city and county agencies, and universities in areas such as organization assessment, strategic planning, coaching, leadership, and program assessment and evaluation. She serves as a consultant for group relations conferences in the United States, Europe, and Asia. She has received $20 million in grant funding.

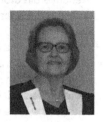

Linda Christensen, EdD, JD, RN is a nurse-educator-administrator-lawyer. She has more than 40 years of experience in nursing education, ranging from teaching nursing assistant classes at a community college to teaching graduate nursing students. During her years as an education administrator, she served as program director (for various levels of nursing), dean of nursing, and vice president of academic affairs. As a lawyer, she has served as a civil litigator, in-house attorney, and legal writing instructor. She is a frequent guest speaker on legal issues, with a particular focus on nursing education and the law. Dr. Christensen has authored various chapters on legal issues in nursing and was co-editor of NLN's *Scope of Practice for Academic Nurse Educators and Academic Clinical Nurse Educators, Third Edition.* She is currently the chief legal officer for the NLN.

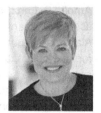

Susan Gross Forneris, PhD, RN, CNE, CHSE-A, FAAN is a former professor of nursing at St. Catherine University, St. Paul, Minnesota and is currently the director for the NLN Center for Innovation in Education Excellence, Washington, DC. Selected for inclusion in the 2010 inaugural group of NLN Simulation Leaders, she has been working in the field of clinical simulation since 2003. She continues to be instrumental in the design and implementation of NLN faculty development resources focused on the pedagogy of teaching and learning. She uses her expertise in curriculum and teaching/learning strategies, with an emphasis in simulation and debriefing, to enhance the knowledge and skills of nurse educators. Her research and publications focus on the development and use of reflective teaching strategies to enhance critical thinking. She co-authored *Critical Conversations: The NLN Guide for Teaching Thinking* and, most recently, *Critical Conversations: From Monologue to Dialogue.*

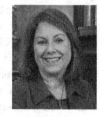

Karen Frith, PhD, RN, NEC-BC, CNE earned a BSN from Auburn University, an MSN with a specialty in Nursing Administration from the University of North Carolina in Greensboro, and a PhD in Nursing with a concentration in Nursing Education from Georgia State University. She is board certified as a Nurse Executive, Advanced by the American Nurses Credentialing Center and certified as a Nurse Educator by the NLN. Dr. Frith worked in critical care for 10 years before moving into an academic role. She has enjoyed 25 years of teaching in universities and is currently the associate dean for Graduate Programs at the University of Alabama in Huntsville. Dr. Frith has a notable publication record of more than 60 peer-reviewed journal articles, 15 book chapters, and two books. Her scholarship focuses in two areas: informatics to improve patient outcomes regarding healthcare delivery and educational technology to improve outcomes in higher education. Dr. Frith writes the Emerging Technologies column for *Nursing Education Perspectives* and serves on the editorial board for the same journal.

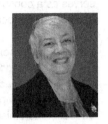

Judith A. Halstead, PhD, RN, CNE, FAAN, ANEF was the founding executive director of the National League for Nursing Commission for Nursing Education Accreditation in Washington, DC, a position she held from 2014-2021. Dr. Halstead holds the rank of professor emerita at Indiana University School of Nursing, Indianapolis, Indiana. She has more than 40 years of experience in nursing education with expertise in online education, nurse educator competencies, interprofessional education, and program evaluation. She is co-editor of the widely referenced book on nursing education, *Teaching in Nursing: A Guide for Faculty,* now in its sixth edition, and is the recipient of numerous awards including the MNRS Advancement of Science Award for the Nursing Education Research Section and the Sigma Theta Tau International Elizabeth Russell Belford Excellence in Education Award. She is a Fellow in the NLN Academy of Nursing Education and the American Academy of Nursing. She served as the president of the NLN from 2011 to 2013.

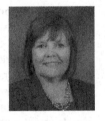

Amelia S. Lanz, EdD, RN, CNE is a clinical assistant professor and associate dean for undergraduate programs at the University of Alabama in Huntsville College of Nursing. She served as coordinator for curriculum and instruction in the College of Nursing before assuming the associate dean's post. Her nursing experience spans more than 30 years, 15 of which have been devoted to classroom and clinical instruction. She received an EdD in Instructional Leadership in Nursing Education from the University of Alabama in 2016 and is an NLN certified nurse educator. She is also an NLN LEAD Fellow. She has presented her work and successfully published manuscripts centered on nursing education. Her five years of work in administration has required an extensive focus on nursing student retention and recruitment, and her latest work focuses on the collaborative development of innovative programs to decrease attrition.

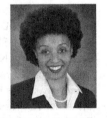

Jacquelyn McMillian-Bohler, PhD, CNM, CNE received a BSN from the University of North Carolina at Greensboro, an MSN in Nurse-Midwifery from Vanderbilt University, and a PhD in Nursing Education from Villanova University. Currently an assistant clinical professor at Duke University School of Nursing, she teaches health promotion and perinatal nursing in the accelerated BSN (ABSN) and master's degree programs. Passionate about students' learning and helping others achieve excellence in teaching, Dr. McMillian-Bohler's program of research aims to identify how master teachers create powerful learning experiences for students. She has presented nationally, regionally, and locally on the topics related to faculty development, and has published articles exploring the master teacher concept and teaching strategies, as well as addressing racial bias. She also is passionate about global health and has precepted nursing students in China, South America, and the Philippines. As a certified nurse-midwife, Dr. McMillian-Bohler provided full scope women's health care in Charleston, South Carolina, Nashville, Tennessee, and Louisville, Kentucky. Her notable recognitions include the Alumni Award for Clinical Achievement from Vanderbilt University, the American College of Nurse-Midwives Vanderbilt Nurse-Midwifery Faculty of the Year, the Kentucky African American Nurses Association Educator of the Year Award, a research award from the Alpha Nu Chapter (Villanova University) of Sigma Theta Tau, and an ABSN Faculty Excellence Teaching Award at Duke University School of Nursing.

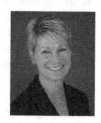

Angela M. McNelis, PhD, RN, CNE, FAAN, ANEF is a leader, scholar, and educator transforming nursing education through her evidence-based research, landmark studies, pedagogical innovations, and dissemination of results locally, nationally, and internationally. Her leadership and work advance the science by developing evidence to direct transformative changes in education across pre-licensure, graduate, and doctoral education. She is at the forefront of national efforts to transform nursing education so that new nurses from entry to advanced levels are prepared for practice. Over her 20-year academic career, she provided leadership on a series of grants focused on exploring and developing models to improve clinical and didactic education in undergraduate and graduate programs; increasing the number and diversity of advanced practice psychiatric mental health nursing students and graduates; improving the practice skills of advanced practice nurses and social workers to screen and intervene with clients who have substance use disorders; increasing the prevalence and rigor of interprofessional education at all levels; and understanding barriers and facilitators to increasing the number of faculty in schools of nursing nationally. She truly is a leading voice for transforming nursing education scholarship through her significant and sustained record of publications, national and international conference presentations, teaching, and leadership. Her body of work that generates nursing knowledge on best practices in teaching and learning advance the quality of education for nurses at all levels and their preparedness to deliver safe, high-quality care and education.

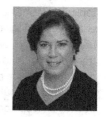

Joanne Noone, PhD, RN, CNE, FAAN, ANEF is an AB Youmans Spaulding Distinguished Professor and campus associate dean at the Ashland Campus of the Oregon Health & Science University School of Nursing. Dr. Noone has more than three decades of experience teaching nursing in associate degree and baccalaureate programs, RN-to-BS completion programs, and master's and doctoral programs. She currently teaches in the Masters in Nursing Education program at OHSU in which three of the courses she teaches are certified by Quality Matters, meeting national standards for best practices in online education. Dr. Noone received her PhD in nursing from the University of Hawaii in 2003. She has been certified since 2009 in nursing education by the NLN and was inducted as a Fellow in the NLN Academy of Nursing Education in 2017 and the American Academy of Nursing in 2018. Dr. Noone's contributions to nursing education aim to promote health equity through learning activities that prepare nurses to care for diverse populations and strategies to improve nursing workforce diversity. In relation to the latter focus, she developed a model for undergraduate nursing programs that focuses on recruitment, enrollment, retention, and graduation of diverse students, an initiative that has had an impact on improved representation of underrepresented minority graduates in associated nursing programs.

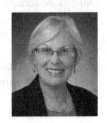

Marilyn H. Oermann, PhD, RN, FAAN, ANEF is the Thelma M. Ingles Professor of Nursing at Duke University School of Nursing, Durham, North Carolina. She is the editor-in-chief of *Nurse Educator* and the *Journal of Nursing Care Quality*. Dr. Oermann is the author/co-author of 23 books, more than 195 articles in peer-reviewed journals, and many editorials, chapters, and other types of publications. Her current books are (1) *Evaluation and Testing in Nursing Education*; (2) *Writing for Publication in Nursing*; (3) *Clinical Teaching Strategies in Nursing*; (4) *Teaching in Nursing and Role of the Educator: The Complete Guide to Best Practice in Teaching, Evaluation, and Curriculum Development*; and (5) *A Systematic Approach to Assessment and Evaluation of Nursing Programs*. She also edited six volumes of the *Annual Review of Nursing Education*. Dr. Oermann is a Fellow in both the American Academy of Nursing and the NLN's Academy of Nursing Education. She received the NLN Award for Excellence in Nursing Education Research, the Sigma Theta Tau International Elizabeth Russell Belford Award for Excellence in Education, the American Association of Colleges of Nursing Scholarship of Teaching and Learning Excellence Award, the Margaret Comerford Freda Award for Editorial Leadership in Nursing from the International Academy of Nursing Editors, and the NLN President's Award.

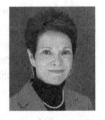

Barbara Patterson, PhD, RN, FAAN, ANEF is a distinguished professor, director of the PhD program, and associate dean for scholarship and inquiry in the School of Nursing at Widener University in Chester, Pennsylvania. She is also the distinguished scholar in the NLN/Chamberlain Center for Advancing the Science of Nursing Education. Dr. Patterson has chaired more than 50 PhD dissertations, many of which addressed nursing education topics, and she has presented and published extensively in nursing education, specifically in the areas of evidence-based teaching, veterans' academic transitions, and leadership in nursing education. Her passion is in the generation and translation of evidence for nursing education practice. She has served as faculty and mentor for novice nurse educators in the Nurse Faculty Leadership Academies of Sigma Theta Tau International focusing on leadership development. Dr. Patterson was chair of NLN's Research Review Panel from 2012 to 2015 and continues as staff liaison to review nursing education research grants. Dr. Patterson is the editor-in-chief for *Nursing Education Perspectives*.

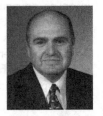

Demetrius James Porche, DNS, PhD, PCC, FACHE, FAANP, FAAN, ANEF is professor and dean of Louisiana State University Health-New Orleans School of Nursing. He also holds an appointment in the School of Public Health at Louisiana State University Health-New Orleans. He received his undergraduate BSN from Nicholls State University, his MSN and DNS from

Louisiana State University Medical Center, and completed family nurse practitioner post-graduate coursework at Concordia University in Wisconsin. Dr. Porche earned a doctor of philosophy degree from Capella University in Organization and Management with a specialization in Leadership. He is certified as a clinical specialist in community health nursing and as a family nurse practitioner, and he is board certified in healthcare by the American College of Healthcare Executives. Dr. Porche was inducted as a Fellow in the American College of Healthcare Executives, the American Academy of Nurse Practitioners, and the American Academy of Nursing.

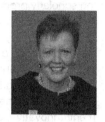

M. Elaine Tagliareni, EdD, RN, CNE, FAAN is a professor and dean of the School of Nursing at the MGH Institute of Health Professions (IHP) in Boston. She joined MGH IHP after serving as a chief program officer at the NLN from 2010 through 2017. For more than 25 years prior to her appointment at the NLN, Dr. Tagliareni was a professor of nursing and the Independence Foundation chair in Community Health Nursing Education at the Community College of Philadelphia. She has a long history of organizational leadership, including service as president of the NLN from 2007 to 2009, as well as leading grant-funded and other national initiatives to support models that increase the academic progression of all nursing graduates and provide patient-centric care for older adults and their caregivers.

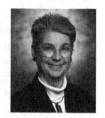

Theresa M. "Terry" Valiga, EdD, RN, CNE, FAAN, ANEF received her bachelor's degree from Trenton State College and her master of education and doctor of education degrees (both in Nursing Education) from Teachers College, Columbia University. She is professor emerita at the Duke University School of Nursing, having served as director of their Institute for Educational Excellence and chair of their Division of Clinical Systems and Analytics until her retirement in August 2017. Terry also served as the chief program officer at the NLN and held faculty and administrative positions in five universities over a 26-year period: Trenton State College, Seton Hall, Georgetown, Villanova, and Fairfield Universities, where she was the dean of the School of Nursing for four years. Dr. Valiga has completed research related to student learning, cognitive/intellectual development, curriculum design, leadership development, student perspectives of excellent teachers, and student evaluations of courses and teachers. She has received grants to support scholarly endeavors, published extensively on a variety of leadership and education-related topics, co-authored five books (including co-editing/co-authoring the NLN's 2009 book, *Achieving Excellence in Nursing Education,* and co-authoring a book on leadership that is now in its sixth edition), presented papers and workshops at national and international conferences, served as a consultant to many schools of nursing inside and outside the United States, and provided leadership in several professional organizations. She has received the NLN's Outstanding Leadership in Nursing Education Award and Sigma's Elizabeth Russell Belford Founders Award for Excellence in Nursing Education and is a Fellow in the American Academy of Nursing and the NLN's Academy of Nursing Education.

Foreword

Nurse educators are known for their ability to meet the moment in the face of change by adapting teaching-learning strategies to engage each student, revising curricula to respond to evolving healthcare and community needs, and maintaining scholarly productivity. Although faculty continually strive for excellence, our work is not always recognized. The *Hallmarks of Excellence in Nursing Education©* serve as a guide to pursuing, attaining, and recognizing excellence, and they offer a framework in which to embed our work.

The editors and contributors to this landmark book have significantly updated the original framework for excellence to include eight interlocking Hallmarks: Engaged Students; Diverse, Well-Prepared Faculty; Culture of Continuous Quality Improvement; Innovative, Evidence-based Curriculum; Innovative, Evidence-based Approaches to Facilitate and Evaluate Learning; Resources to Support Program Goal Attainment; Commitment to Pedagogical Scholarship; and Effective Institutional and Professional Leadership. The revised Hallmarks and Indicators were derived from a survey of a broad base of nurse educators and represent the current state of the science that underlies our work.

In the chapters that describe the evidence base for each Hallmark (Chapters 3 through 10), readers will find the necessary resources to set the path for excellence at their school and in their own practice. Using the Indicators, the questions educators can use to reflect on the concept of excellence, and the self-assessment guide, administrators and faculty can identify areas of strength and those needing improvement. Readers will find the Hallmarks helpful in curriculum planning, promoting student engagement, guiding policy development, seeking awards and recognition, and providing a framework for scholarly work.

The editors and contributors invite you to embark on the journey of recognizing, seeking, and attaining excellence and distinction in nursing education. Let our light continue to shine!

Diane M. Billings, EdD, RN, FAAN, ANEF
Chancellor's Professor Emeritus
Indiana University School of Nursing, Indianapolis

Preface

The ultimate goal for every school/college is to strive for excellence to achieve distinction so as to set one's school/college apart from others because of its dedication to quality education and programming. This cannot be achieved without a diverse, well-prepared faculty; engaged students; an innovative, evidence-based curriculum and approaches to facilitate and evaluate learning; resources to support goal attainment and growth; a commitment to scholarship, particularly as it relates to education; a commitment to continuous quality improvement; and effective leadership.

Achieving Distinction in Nursing Education is based on the National League for Nursing's (NLN's) *Hallmarks of Excellence in Nursing Education Model©* (see Appendix A). which depicts the eight core elements required to achieve excellence and distinction in nursing education. Each Hallmark and its accompanying Indicators help schools/colleges assess their strengths and identify the areas that need further development to achieve excellence and distinction.

Chapters 1 and 2 provide an analysis of the concepts of *excellence* and *distinction*, as well as the historical context regarding the development of the Hallmarks. Chapters 3 through 10 each address one of the core elements of the Hallmarks; on the opening page of each of these chapters, a visual depiction of the relevant component of the model is presented in order to highlight the importance of this element but also to remind all of us that it is only one piece in attaining the ultimate goal of excellence in nursing education. In each chapter, evidence is provided to support the relevance of the Hallmark and its Indicators, and exemplars are provided throughout the book to demonstrate how distinction can be attained. Finally, the last chapter addresses key initiatives that the NLN has in place to support faculty and nursing programs as they pursue excellence and distinction.

This book features contributions from 15 recognized experts and leaders in the field of nursing education, administration, and research. These contributors have experience working with all types of nursing programs including LPN/LVN, associate degree, baccalaureate, master's, and doctoral (PhD and DNP), and they have helped shape our thinking about nursing education through their scholarly work, publications, presentations, consultations, and service in professional associations.

It is our hope that the discussions in this book will inspire and challenge you personally and professionally to invest in yourself and your school/college as you advance in your quest to achieve excellence and distinction in nursing education.

Marsha Adams and Terry Valiga, Editors

Acknowledgments

We wish to acknowledge several individuals whose contributions were significant in the production of this book. First of all, our sincere thanks go to the National League for Nursing (NLN) for their wisdom regarding the need to prepare a book that provides updated perspectives on excellence and distinction in nursing education, as well as on the *Hallmarks of Excellence in Nursing Education©*. We are grateful to Dr. Beverly Malone for writing the "Reflections from the NLN President and CEO" piece that introduces the book and to Dr. Diane Billings for writing the "Foreword" to the book; both individuals are accomplished and highly regarded in the nursing education community, and their willingness to be part of this endeavor is very much appreciated.

We also wish to give public acknowledgment to Dr. Elaine Tagliareni, who worked closely with us throughout the process of updating the Hallmarks. She was instrumental in collaborating to develop, launch, and analyze responses to the survey that is described in Chapter 2, as well as revising the Hallmarks themselves and the visual model that shows their relation to excellence.

To all those NLN members who responded to the survey and provided thoughtful comments about the relevance of, areas of duplication in, and "gaps" in the Hallmarks that had been developed in 2005, we offer our deep thanks. It is through this kind of collegial support that the current Hallmarks were refined to be more reflective of contemporary practices and, therefore, more valuable to the nursing education community.

Finally, we wish to acknowledge the invaluable contributions of those who authored chapters for this book. We are most fortunate to include the perspectives and suggestions of these outstanding leaders in nursing education and are confident that their expertise will be valued by nursing faculty.

Marsha Adams and Terry Valiga, Editors

Contents

List of Tables and Boxes

1

Achieving Distinction in Nursing Education by Continually Pursuing Excellence

Theresa M. "Terry" Valiga, EdD, RN, CNE, FAAN, ANEF

INTRODUCTION

Distinction in nursing education. What is it? Why is it important? And how do we achieve it? All of these questions are critical for nurse educators to address, particularly as the context for our pre-licensure, registered nurse-to-bachelor of science in nursing (RN-to-BSN), and graduate programs change rapidly and the demands for relevance in higher education increase. This book takes on the challenge of discussing these questions and offers the nursing education community research findings, insights, and strategies to address them.

THE CONCEPTS OF DISTINCTION AND EXCELLENCE

Distinction, or *distinctive*, is a word often used to describe some person, thing, or accomplishment that is notable. It is used to describe an individual or organization that is set apart from others because of unique accomplishments or the level of excellence that has been achieved. It is a term synonymous with words like *first-rate*, *great*, *perfect*, or *preeminent* and, obviously, suggests something that takes concerted effort and dedication to achieve. Interestingly, Founding Father John Adams asserted that human beings are driven by what he called "the passion for distinction" (Kronman, 2019, p. 32).

The continual pursuit of excellence can be thought of as a means to achieve distinction, but what does this concept mean? *Excellence* has been defined in many ways, including the following: "striving to be the very best you can be in everything you do—not because some teacher or parent or other 'authority' figure pushes you to do it, but because you cannot imagine functioning in any other way" (Grossman & Valiga, 2021, p. 255). In other words, a commitment to excellence is a value that becomes part of the DNA of an individual or organization and involves "setting high standards . . ., holding . . . to those standards despite challenges or pressures to reduce or lower them, and not being satisfied with anything less than the very best" (Grossman & Valiga, 2021, p. 255).

Individuals and organizations that pursue excellence will not settle for mediocrity, resist change, or accept that the current state is necessarily the best. Instead, they will be willing to invest the time, energy, and resources needed to change practices based on evidence, take risks to implement innovative approaches, and create environments that support and encourage a questioning mind and spirit of inquiry for all members of the community.

PURSUING EXCELLENCE AND ATTAINING DISTINCTION: RELEVANCE TO NURSING EDUCATION

In nursing education, faculty may assume that state board approval and even accreditation are signs of excellence and distinction, but those assumptions need to be challenged. While both designations are important – state board approval is needed to even exist as a program, and accreditation is an indication of successful review of a program's quality by peers – neither particularly sets one program or school apart from others. In essence, both designations convey that (1) the school's curricula make sense and are appropriate to help learners achieve specified outcomes, (2) the school has adequate resources (i.e., faculty, staff, equipment, technology, classroom and laboratory learning spaces, library holdings, clinical placements, etc.) to implement the program, and (3) the school regularly examines its processes and outcomes and uses the data gained from such self-reviews to make needed improvements.

Schools that strive for excellence and distinction, however, expect more than these core standards. They expect that **students** are more than passive learners who pass courses and the licensing or certification exam but, instead, are actively engaged in the learning process, exhibit enthusiasm for learning, are open to new ideas and diverse opinions, and evolve as leaders and scholars who will help shape the future of our profession. These schools expect that **faculty** are innovative, challenge traditional approaches to teaching and evaluation, have some degree of expertise as educators, and are encouraged to embrace and lead change.

Schools that strive for excellence and distinction expect that their **academic leaders** create and sustain healthy work environments, promote civility, and set high expectations for performance. These schools expect that curricula are innovative and designed to promote cultural sensitivity, foster interprofessional collaboration, help students develop strong critical thinking and clinical judgment skills, and enhance learners' identity formation as nurses, leaders, and scholars. Additionally, efforts at such schools are consistently directed to embrace innovative, evidence-based approaches to **facilitate and evaluate learning**.

All of these elements – and more – are clearly articulated in the *Hallmarks of Excellence in Nursing Education*© (National League for Nursing [NLN], 2020) and discussed thoroughly in this book. But why should schools of nursing attend to the Hallmarks and use them for program development, student and faculty recruitment, resource development, and policy formulation? One simple response to that question is, "Because excellence begets excellence." This concept was supported by findings from studies reported by Curtin as long ago as 1990; these studies showed that on units where excellence is the norm, nurses strive to achieve the high level of performance demonstrated by their peers, but on units where practice is poor or mediocre, nurses and others accept the status quo and do not make efforts to improve. In essence, then, when individuals are in an environment that expects and supports excellence – and strives to attain distinction – it becomes contagious and, sooner or later, even the most recalcitrant members of the community also are learning, growing, trying new things, challenging the status quo, and pushing to do their very best. Communities such as these are more likely to attract highly qualified students and distinguished faculty, have lower turnover rates, garner greater respect and admiration from colleagues, and be rewarded for their innovation and accomplishments.

Another reason to continually strive for excellence relates to the purpose of higher education. In a thoughtful book entitled *The Assault on American Excellence*, Kronman (2019, p. 13) notes that "our colleges and universities are devoted to the shaping of souls as distinct from the transmission of skills" (p. 13), and they have a responsibility to foster "tolerance for ambiguity and dissonance . . . [that] encourages doubt and self-reflection and breaks the tendency to go along with what 'everyone is saying'" (p. 19). This former dean of the Yale School of Law asserts that "human excellence . . . is valuable for its own sake and as an aid to the independent-mindedness on which the health of our democracy depends" (p. 15); he suggests that faculty strive to provide students with an education in human excellence that increases their chances of becoming excellent human beings. Surely, nurse educators desire to do more than merely transmit content or develop clinical skills. To prepare our students to function effectively in the chaotic, uncertain, ever-changing environments of today and tomorrow they, instead, design curricula, employ teaching and evaluation strategies, create environments, and engage in continuous quality improvement efforts that serve to help students develop as excellent human beings – who know who they *are* – as well as capable nurses – who know what they *do*. Continually striving for excellence, therefore, clearly is relevant in nursing education.

As noted by Aristotle, "We are what we repeatedly do. Excellence is not an act, but a habit." In other words, the pursuit of excellence is not something one does now and then; it is continuous and, as stated earlier, is part of the DNA of an individual or organization. And this pursuit helps avoid two grave dangers: the loss of esteem for human greatness and the "tyranny of the majority [where] the habit of independent thinking is on the decline [and individuals] tend increasingly to be steered by public opinion instead" (Kronman, 2019, p. 39).

EXCELLENCE AND DISTINCTION VERSUS PERFECTION

Oftentimes, the notions of excellence and distinction are rejected because it is assumed that they imply perfection . . . and perfection is impossible to attain, particularly in complex, multifaceted, and constantly changing entities like nursing education. But such an assumption is unwarranted because pursuing excellence and achieving distinction does not mean perfection. The words of former Green Bay Packers Coach Vince Lombardi are helpful in understanding the relationship among these notions. Lombardi wisely told his players, "Perfection is not attainable, but if we chase perfection, we can catch excellence."

Thus, faculty, deans, directors, and others involved in nursing education need not fear that perfection is expected when discussions of excellence and distinction arise. We are all human, and humans make mistakes. We try and we fail. But that is part of the excellence journey . . . to take the risk of doing something new, different, or innovative . . . possibly failing . . . and learning from that result. A proposal to orient new faculty in a different way than has been in place for years, for example, may reflect findings from a literature review and be successful in another school, but it may not be as successful in your institution because of your culture, resources, or other factors. However, recognizing that the current approach to new faculty orientation is not as effective as it could be is a step toward excellence in and of itself; and the modifications in the proposed approach that are made after careful reflection on a failure are likely to lead to an orientation program that is most appropriate for your environment and well-received by all who participate in it. Thus, the goal is not to be perfect; instead, the goal is to continually pursue excellence and, ultimately, achieve distinction.

STRATEGIES TO PURSUE EXCELLENCE AND ACHIEVE DISTINCTION

There are many ways faculty in a particular school can embark on the journey toward excellence and distinction. One way to begin is to have open discussions about the Hallmarks and the Indicators that accompany each (see Appendix B) . . . what they mean, why and how they are relevant in your situation, and how your school can use them to guide curriculum development, implementation, and evaluation; faculty development; student engagement; policy formulation; partnerships with clinical facilities and the surrounding community; scholarly efforts of students and faculty; staff involvement; and so on. Such discussions can occur at general, program, and/or course faculty meetings where a designated period of time is devoted to a selected Hallmark. They can also occur during committee meetings; for example, the curriculum committee could engage in an in-depth analysis of the Hallmark related to innovative, evidence-based curricula; the faculty affairs committee could do the same in relation to the Hallmarks about a diverse, well-prepared faculty and the commitment to pedagogical scholarship; and the dean's advisory committee could use the Hallmark related to effective, institutional, and professional leadership, as well as the one related to resources to support program goal attainment, to guide formulation of a strategic plan for the school.

Another way in which the Hallmarks and Indicators can be used is by conducting a self-assessment, using the Self-Assessment Checklist included in Appendix C. Faculty, staff, and students could be asked to complete the checklist via an online survey tool, offering comments on where they see strengths and what they think needs to be improved. The survey results could then be compiled – in toto, by Hallmark, and/or by respondent group – reviewed for commonalities across respondent groups, analyzed for trends in areas perceived as strengths and areas where improvements would benefit the school, and discussed by various groups. From this analysis, recommendations could be generated regarding how existing strengths could be built upon as well as the strategies that could be used to address weaker areas. By using the Hallmarks and Indicators in this way, the entire school community is involved, all are reminded of the many positive aspects of the school, recommendations for future initiatives evolve from data, the school is positioned as a leader and model within the larger parent institution, and opportunities could arise for publications and presentations to the broader nursing and higher education communities.

In addition to self-reflection leading to publications and presentations to internal and external audiences, the pursuit of excellence could emerge as an area of scholarship for faculty and/or students. Faculty with expertise in education – and students preparing for such a role – might develop a program of scholarship that addresses the development of instruments to measure excellence, the creation of resources to support it, or the impact of pursuing it on student learning, faculty morale and productivity, clinical partnerships, diversity and inclusion efforts, and reputation. Faculty with expertise in clinical practice, as well as beginning and advanced students, might pursue research that examines practicing nurses' efforts to achieve excellence in patient/family care along with the barriers to such efforts and the factors that support and encourage it. And those with an interest in systems might engage in scholarly activities that address ways in which organizational cultures, mechanisms to encourage civility and inclusion, and policies enhance the pursuit of excellence and attainment of distinction.

Excellence also means being "unwilling to accept the status quo" (Grossman & Valiga, 2021, p. 256). In a discussion directed primarily to academic departments and the role of the chair, dean, or director, Wergin (2003) offered advice that is as relevant today as it was shortly after the turn of the century. He asserted that "the most useful way to build and sustain a culture of excellence is to create a culture of critical reflection and continuous improvement" (p. xiii). These concepts are evident in the Hallmarks related to **continuous quality improvement** and **effective institutional and professional leadership**, and they warrant serious attention by schools pursuing excellence and hoping to achieve distinction.

Finally, in their annual evaluations, faculty could be asked to discuss the particular Hallmark(s) they addressed during the past year and the one(s) they plan to address in the coming year. For example, relatively new faculty members may choose to focus their energies on the Hallmark about **engaged students**, designing, implementing, and evaluating various ways to promote a spirit of inquiry among students; helping them be creative and innovative; and thinking of themselves as leaders and scholars as well as clinicians. In subsequent years, these faculty may choose to focus on developing **innovative, evidence-based approaches to evaluating learning** in ways that acknowledge the uniqueness and diversity of learners. And further along in their career development, faculty may choose to explore ways in which the **curriculum** could be more flexible to meet student learning needs and still maintain its integrity, or to develop their skills as pedagogical scholars.

In summary, there are many strategies that individuals and schools of nursing can employ to address the pursuit of excellence and attainment of distinction and, perhaps, advance our understanding of these important concepts.

THE COMPLEXITY OF EXCELLENCE AND DISTINCTION

It should be apparent from this discussion that excellence is a complex concept, and achieving excellence in nursing education calls for multifaceted efforts. This complexity is depicted in the NLN's *Hallmarks of Excellence in Nursing Education Model©* (see Appendix A).

A school of nursing, for example, can have a large, state-of-the-art, fully equipped lab, but if faculty do not know how to use that resource to its fullest extent in order to facilitate student learning, it is not likely that excellence will be achieved. Likewise, 100 percent of the faculty in a school might be doctorally prepared, but if those faculty do not know how to design curricula that are internally consistent and appropriate for the identified learning outcomes, or if they do not know how to engage in scholarly teaching that effectively meets the learning needs of the diverse student population, achieving excellence is unlikely. Similarly, a school can have a comprehensive program evaluation plan and collect extensive amounts of data from students, faculty, staff, and clinical partners, but excellence will not be achieved if those data are not studied seriously and used to make improvements in the school's culture, curriculum, approaches to facilitating and evaluating learning, relationships with clinical partners, and so on. In essence, faculty need to see that all elements of the model are attended to if the goal is to continually pursue excellence.

Although pursuing and achieving excellence in nursing education is complex and multifaceted, schools often move to a level of distinction in one area or another. For example, some schools have a deep and abiding *commitment to pedagogical scholarship*, where many faculty – and even students – are engaged in scholarly activities designed to advance the science of nursing education; such a school comes to be known and respected in the nursing education community for its scholarly contributions, faculty are sought out by colleagues for consultation, and the school achieves designation as an NLN Center of Excellence in Nursing Education™ in the category of "Advancing the Science of Nursing Education" (see Chapter 11 for more details on the NLN's Centers of Excellence program).

Distinction might also be achieved in the area of *innovative, evidence-based approaches to facilitate and evaluate learning* when faculty continuously design, implement, and evaluate the effectiveness of new ways to fully engage students in the learning process, disseminate those efforts widely, earn awards and honors from professional associations for this work, and are showcased within their own institution as a model of excellence in teaching and learning. And yet another school might achieve distinction for the way in which it *uses resources to support program goal attainment*, particularly through the creation of innovative connections with clinical partners.

CONCLUSION

The concepts of excellence and distinction are complex, and neither outcome is easily achieved. Indeed, excellence is attained only through the concerted efforts of all members of the academic community, and a school can achieve distinction only when its students, faculty, and curricula are acknowledged for their innovation, focus, and productive interactions.

This book provides readers with an analysis of each of the eight NLN Hallmarks, providing evidence to support the inclusion of each as a key element in the journey toward excellence and offering ideas regarding what schools can do to achieve each Hallmark. Readers are challenged to carefully review the Hallmarks and Indicators (Appendix B), use the Self-Assessment Checklist (Appendix C), and engage in serious reflection on the strengths of their own schools, as well as areas where improvement is needed to achieve excellence. Readers are then challenged to consider how their strengths can be used to achieve distinction in a specific area, particularly through those programs offered by the NLN – Centers of Excellence program, certification of nurse educators, and the Academy of Nursing Education – all of which are described in Chapter 11.

"Some say that in our society as a whole, and in nursing in particular, we have for too long accepted the mundane, promoted the average, and rewarded the mediocre" (Valiga, 2009, p. 4). Those schools that make a commitment to pursue excellence and, ultimately, achieve distinction are not likely to promote the average and reward the mediocre. But they are likely to find that faculty are energized by the journey, students and alumni are more fully engaged in the life of the school, the nursing program is held in higher esteem by institutional administrators and colleagues in other disciplines, graduates are highly respected and sought after by employers, all members of the community accomplish great things, productivity is increased, and the school community is a vibrant, healthy, empowering one. Such outcomes would seem to make the pursuit of excellence well worthwhile.

References

Curtin, L. (1990). The excellence within (Editorial Opinion). *Nursing Management, 21* (10), 7.

Grossman, S. C., & Valiga, T. M. (2021). *The new leadership challenge: Creating the future of nursing* (6th ed.). F.A. Davis.

Kronman, A. (2019). *The assault on American excellence*. Free Press.

National League for Nursing. (2020). *Hallmarks of excellence in nursing education*. http://www.nln.org/professional-development-programs/teaching-resources/hallmarks-of-excellence

Valiga, T. M. (2009). Excellence in nursing education: An introduction. In M. H. Adams & T. M. Valiga (Eds.), *Achieving excellence in nursing education* (pp. 1–7). National League for Nursing.

Wergin, J. F. (2003). *Departments that work: Building and sustaining cultures of excellence in academic programs*. Anker.

2

History of the Hallmarks of Excellence in Nursing Education

Marsha Howell Adams, PhD, RN, CNE, FAAN, ANEF

INTRODUCTION

The *Hallmarks of Excellence in Nursing Education©* are "characteristics or traits that serve to define a level of outstanding performance or service" (Adams & Valiga, 2009, p. 11). These Hallmarks challenge schools/colleges of nursing to continually change and improve as they strive to be the very best. The concepts of distinction and excellence are defined and discussed in Chapter 1, and a visual representation of the current National League for Nursing (NLN) *Hallmarks of Excellence in Nursing Education Model©* (NLN, 2020b) is provided. Striving for excellence was the major focus of the original book, *Achieving Excellence in Nursing Education* (Adams & Valiga, 2009); the primary focus of this book extends that focus and challenges faculty to go even one step farther to envision how striving for excellence in nursing education can help lead an organization toward achieving distinction as a school/college of nursing and how using the NLN Hallmarks (NLN, 2020a) serve to guide faculty on that journey. This chapter describes how the Hallmarks were developed initially (NLN, 2004) and how they have been refined (NLN, 2020a) to better reflect the present and the future.

INITIAL DEVELOPMENT OF THE HALLMARKS OF EXCELLENCE

In 2001, the NLN created the Nursing Education Advisory Council (NEAC), whose purpose was to provide leadership that creates dramatic change for nursing education quality and standards. One of the task groups formed under the auspices of NEAC was the Task Group on Nursing Education Standards (Adams & Valiga, 2009, p. 11).

Members of the task group possessed expertise in nursing education and represented all types of nursing education programs. As they began their work in the spring of 2002, task group members were charged with the following (Adams & Valiga, 2009, p. 11):

▸ Conduct a comprehensive literature review of the concept of education standards, as well as existing standards in nursing, related fields, and higher education in general.

> Analyze these standards for their relevance to nursing education in the 21st century.
> Identify gaps in existing standards relative to current nursing practice expectations.
> Create an annotated bibliography of significant literature.
> Formulate a set of nursing education standards that is accompanied by a glossary of significant terms.
> Present this document at an NLN Educational Summit.
> Outline a strategy for effective dissemination of the standards to NLN members and other stakeholders for review and comment.
> Revise/Refine the standards based on feedback.
> Prepare the final standards for publication and dissemination.

To complement the work of the task group, the NLN sponsored a Think Tank on Nursing Education Standards. This group of thought leaders in nursing education, nursing practice, and higher education provided guidance regarding the formulation, dissemination, and identification of strategies to continually review the standards/Hallmarks toward which all educational programs in nursing should strive. Such work would challenge programs to be innovative, create empowering environments, and support evidence-based teaching. Individuals representing the following organizations participated in the think tank and formulated significant recommendations for future work: American Association of Colleges of Nursing, American Association of Colleges of Pharmacy, American Association of Community Colleges, Commission on Graduates of Foreign Nursing Schools, National Council of State Boards of Nursing, National League for Nursing Accrediting Commission, National Nursing Staff Development Organization, National Organization of Associate Degree Nursing, and National Organization of Nurse Practitioner Faculties, as well as the NLN itself (Adams & Valiga, 2009, p. 12).

The Think Tank and the Nursing Education Standards Task Group conducted a comprehensive literature review that focused on standards, the relevance of standard setting to education, the relationship between educational standards and accreditation criteria, and the impact of standards on educational practices. Annotated bibliographies were generated by task group members and uploaded to a comprehensive database created by the NLN. Based on this information, the Hallmarks were developed, reviewed by both groups, and refined (Adams & Valiga, 2009, p. 12).

The Hallmarks were presented to nurse educators attending the NLN Educational Summit in 2002 and again in 2003. During both presentations, feedback was sought; after each dialogue session, the document was further refined.

Despite this valuable input, the task group wanted to obtain feedback from the broader nursing community to "vet" the Hallmarks and stimulate discussion among many faculty groups (Adams & Valiga, 2009, p. 12). Therefore, immediately following the 2003 Summit, a survey was developed and posted to the NLN website, and all faculty and deans/directors in the NLN's database at that time (approximately 10,000 individuals) were invited to respond. The survey was composed of a demographic section, 31 Hallmarks, and 84 Indicators. A glossary also was provided that defined key terms used in the survey. Respondents were asked to indicate whether they agreed or disagreed with each Hallmark and each Indicator and to suggest revisions/refinements to any or all of the items in the comment section that was available for each Hallmark and group of Indicators (Adams & Valiga, 2009, p. 12).

In total, 242 individuals responded to the survey. Although this number was low, the task group was pleased with this response rate due to the length of the survey and the type of thoughtful responses it generated. For 29 of the 31 Hallmarks, 80.6 percent to 95.8 percent of those responding agreed that they reflected a level of excellence, were relevant to all types of programs, and should be retained. The Hallmark addressing "partnerships" in relation to the teaching/learning/evaluation process received a 76.8 percent level of support, and only 63.4 percent of respondents were in agreement with the Hallmark related to using innovation to "create a preferred future for nursing" (Adams & Valiga, 2009, p. 12).

It was clear to the task group that respondents supported the Hallmarks (NLN, 2004) and believed that they challenged nurse educators to strive toward higher levels of achievement. The broad nursing community, as well as the NLN, therefore, viewed the Hallmarks as a means to promote excellence in nursing education programs (Adams & Valiga, 2009, p. 13). With this documented support, the Hallmarks were widely disseminated, and faculty were encouraged to use them as they designed curricula, developed strategies to facilitate and evaluate learning, and evaluated the effectiveness of the programs they offered.

REFINEMENT OF THE HALLMARKS OF EXCELLENCE

In 2018, the editors and co-authors of *Achieving Excellence in Nursing Education* (Adams & Valiga, 2009) in conjunction with NLN staff decided that in light of how the context for nursing education and practice had changed since the initial document was developed, it was time to refine the *Hallmarks of Excellence in Nursing Education©* (NLN, 2004). When making these refinements, it was especially important to gain insight from nurse educators across the country, so a survey was created requesting participants to reexamine each Hallmark and their Indicators for relevancy. Respondents were also asked to suggest revisions to any Hallmark or Indicator that needed to be clarified or strengthened, or to recommend deletion of a Hallmark or Indicator and provide an explanation for that recommendation.

Participants also were asked to provide feedback regarding whether the Indicators for each Hallmark were appropriate examples to support an understanding of the Hallmark's meaning/intent, and they were invited to suggest "other Indicators" that would be helpful. Table 2-1 provides an example of how Hallmarks and Indicators were addressed on the survey.

The survey was disseminated to four groups – all NLN members, Academy of Nursing Education Fellows (ANEF), NLN Center of Excellence (COE) school deans, and the NLN Civility Action Group – and each was asked to respond to questions about certain Hallmarks. For example, Fellows in the Academy of Nursing Education were asked to respond to Hallmarks related to faculty, curriculum, teaching/learning/evaluation, innovation, and leadership, whereas the NLN Civility Action Group responded to Hallmarks addressing faculty, students, and environment. NLN members had the opportunity to respond to all the Hallmarks.

TABLE 2-1

Example of an Item on the Hallmarks Survey Regarding Faculty

Faculty

HALLMARKS & INDICATORS	SURVEY QUESTIONS
The unique contributions of each faculty member in helping the program achieve its goals are valued, rewarded, and recognized.	Is this Hallmark still relevant? YES NO If you responded YES, does YES NO the Hallmark need to be revised in any way? If you think revisions are needed, please offer suggestions on HOW to revise it. If you think this Hallmark is NO LONGER RELEVANT, please explain.
• Are the unique contributions of faculty whose expertise is in education valued, rewarded, and recognized? • Are the unique contributions of faculty whose expertise is in clinical practice valued, rewarded, and recognized? • Are the unique contributions of faculty whose expertise is in research valued, rewarded, and recognized? • Are mechanisms in place that ensure faculty contributions in each area (i.e., teaching, clinical practice, or research) are valued, rewarded, and recognized as significant in helping the program achieve its goals? • Do criteria for faculty reward and recognition acknowledge that one's expertise and significant professional contributions may be in education, practice, or research?	Do you think the five Indicators for YES NO this Hallmark provide examples that help faculty understand its meaning/intent? Feel free to suggest other "Indicators" that would be helpful to faculty.

A total of 823 responses were received: 657 from NLN members, 69 from Fellows in the Nursing Education Academy, 95 from COE school deans, and two from Civility Action Group members. Relevancy of Hallmarks based on survey results is reported in Table 2-2. It was clear that all groups found the existing Hallmarks relevant, but felt that there also was some redundancy. This resulted in the deletion of the Hallmarks addressing Innovation and Environment and distribution of information from both of these areas across other Hallmarks and Indicators.

Based on feedback from respondents, the names of Hallmark categories were reviewed and revised for clarity. Table 2-3 shows the original and revised names of those categories.

TABLE 2-2

Relevancy of Hallmarks: Selective Group Survey Results

Hallmarks of Excellence in Nursing Education© (NLN, 2004)	Relevancy by the NLN Membership (% Agreement)	Relevancy by Other Groups Responding (% Agreement)
Students	95.4%	COE Schools: 92.6%
Faculty	96.4%	ANEF: 98.6%
Continuous Quality Improvement	99.4%	COE Schools: 96.9%
Curriculum	97.9%	ANEF: 88.5%
Facilitating & Evaluating Learning	97.5%	ANEF: 91.3%
Resources	98.25%	COE Schools: 95.7%
Innovation*	96.1%	ANEF: 92.8%
Educational research	96.4%	ANEF: 93.5%
Environment*	98.7%	COE Schools: 93.8%
Leadership	96.7%	ANEF: 91.3%

*Hallmark eventually deleted; Indicators redistributed.

ANEF, Academy of Nursing Education Fellows; COE, Center of Excellence; NLN, National League for Nursing.

TABLE 2-3

Hallmark Category Changes

Then (NLN, 2004) N = 10	Now (NLN, 2020) N = 8
Students	Engaged Students
Faculty	Diverse, Well-Prepared Faculty
Continuous Quality Improvement	A Culture of Continuous Quality Improvement
Curriculum	Innovative, Evidence-Based Curriculum
Teaching/Learning/Evaluation	Innovative, Evidence-Based Approaches to Facilitate and Evaluate Learning
Resources	Resources to Support Program Goal Attainment
Innovation	Deleted
Educational Research	Commitment to Pedagogical Scholarship
Environment	Deleted
Leadership	Effective Institutional and Professional Leadership

NLN, National League for Nursing.

Close scrutiny of participants' survey comments revealed that they consistently identified the following areas as needing more emphasis in the Hallmarks and Indicators: interprofessional education and practice, diversity/inclusivity, faculty clinical practice, leadership, online education, civility, technology/informatics, and mentorship. Table 2-4 provides examples of how the Hallmarks and Indicators for the newly named category *Diverse Well-Prepared Faculty* were refined to address survey participants' recommendations for areas to be enhanced.

Additionally, all Indicators were changed to be open-ended, rather than yes/no, questions so that faculty reviewing them would be challenged to think about their own institution. All refined Hallmarks with their Indicators are included in Appendix B.

In 2005, the *Excellence in Nursing Education Model* (NLN, 2005) was developed to depict, visually, the many areas schools must consider as they strive to achieve excellence in nursing education and the complexity of that concept. The model was designed to be applicable to all types of nursing programs, and the elements included in it were not intended to be exhaustive or all-inclusive. Despite its usefulness, however, the model was flawed in that it did not demonstrate a direct link to the Hallmarks even though the linkage could be implied. To address this flaw, the *Excellence in Nursing Education Model©* (NLN, 2020b) was revised to show the true connection to the Hallmarks, emphasizing the

TABLE 2-4	
Example of Changes for *Diverse, Well-Prepared Faculty* Hallmark and Indicators Based on Survey Results	
Hallmark	**Updated Hallmark**
The faculty complement includes a cadre of individuals who have expertise as educators, clinicians, and as is relevant to the institution's mission and researchers.	**The faculty complement is comprised of diverse individuals who are leaders and/or have expertise in clinical practice, education, interprofessional collaboration, and research/scholarship consistent with the parent institution's mission and vision.**
Indicator	**Updated/New Indicator**
	To what extent does the faculty complement reflect diversity, including race, ethnicity, gender, educational background, and so on?
Does the faculty selection process include specific hiring criteria that deliberately search for candidates whose excellence in education, clinical practice, or research will help create a balanced cadre of full-time faculty?	**To what extent do hiring practices help to create a faculty complement that reflects expertise in education, clinical practice, interprofessional collaboration, and/or research/scholarship?**
Do faculty job responsibility statements specifically address the expert behaviors required for the role of educator, clinician, and researcher?	**To what extent do faculty members' job responsibility statements specifically address the expert behaviors required for the roles of educator, clinician, and researcher/scholar?**

complexity of the educational enterprise and hopefully stimulating the thinking of administrators, faculty, and students related to striving for excellence and achieving distinction in nursing schools/colleges. The model opens the opportunity to welcome distinct perspectives on how schools and programs are meeting the Hallmarks.

CONCLUSION

The journey to develop and refine the NLN *Hallmarks of Excellence in Nursing Education©* (NLN, 2004, NLN, 2020a) is well documented. It is clear through the survey comments that the Hallmarks and Indicators are found to be relevant as well as vital to striving for excellence and achieving distinction. In the chapters that follow, each component of the NLN Hallmarks and the accompanying model (NLN, 2020b) are explored in detail, and evidence is provided to support the importance of the Hallmarks and Indicators. The examples provided serve to demonstrate how a Hallmark can be met when striving for excellence and achieving distinction in nursing education, and the Self-Assessment Checklist provided as Appendix C is offered as a tool to help faculty reflect on their progress toward achieving excellence and distinction.

References

Adams, M., & Valiga, T. (2009). Excellence: Everyone's responsibility. In M. Adams & T. Valiga (Eds.), *Achieving excellence in nursing education* (pp. 9–15). National League for Nursing.

National League for Nursing. (2004). *Hallmarks of excellence in nursing education*. https://www.nln.org/excellence/hallmarks_indicators.htm

National League for Nursing. (2005). *Excellence in nursing education model*. National League for Nursing.

National League for Nursing. (2020a). *Hallmarks of excellence in nursing education*. http://www.nln.org/docs/default-source/default-document-library/hallmarks_of_excellence_2019.pdf?sfvrsn=0

National League for Nursing. (2020b). *Hallmarks of excellence in nursing education model*. http://www.nln.org/professional-development-programs/teaching-resources/hallmarks-of-excellence#:~:text=The%20Hallmarks%20of%20Excellence%C2%A9,and%20institutions%20of%20higher%20learning

3

Engaged Students: Essential to Achieve Distinction in Nursing Education

Joanne Noone, PhD, RN, CNE, FAAN, ANEF

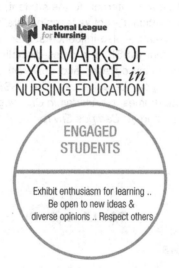

National League *for* **Nursing**

HALLMARKS OF
EXCELLENCE *in*
NURSING EDUCATION

ENGAGED
STUDENTS

Exhibit enthusiasm for learning ..
Be open to new ideas &
diverse opinions .. Respect others

INTRODUCTION

Student engagement is critical not only to academic success in the student's field of study, but it also is vital to promote commitment to lifelong learning and dedication to a professional career. This chapter reviews the key elements of student engagement from the educational and nursing literature, and identifies best practices and strategies that promote student engagement in undergraduate and graduate education. These elements of student engagement are related to student characteristics, to the characteristics of academic environments that promote and support engagement (Harper & Quaye, 2015), to quality learning and academic success (Currey et al., 2015), and to excellence in nursing education.

Student engagement is defined as a dynamic, iterative process of investment, participation, and commitment to learning (Bernard, 2015: Bowcock & Peters, 2016), and it is comprised of behavioral, cognitive, and emotional aspects (Hudson & Carrasco, 2015). *Behavioral aspects* that are associated with student engagement include active participation, attendance, and completion of assignments (Bernard, 2015), as well as collaboration and teamwork (Bowcock & Peters, 2016). *Cognitive aspects* are considered psychological components and include concentration, commitment, sense of purpose, and motivation (Bernard, 2015). *Emotional aspects* of engagement include self-confidence, resilience, and ability to socialize with peers and faculty (Bowcock & Peters, 2016; Johnson, 2015). In fact, a survey of more than 200 undergraduate business majors revealed that peer relationships, faculty-student relationships, and students' sense of purpose have a positive influence on student engagement (Xerri et al., 2018). Undoubtedly, psychological components influence students' engagement in academic activities.

In addition to aspects that are "internal" to the student, the academic environment and the activities that occur within it – active teaching strategies, faculty engagement, and a supportive campus climate – also influence student engagement. The National Survey of Student Engagement (NSSE) is a cross-discipline annual survey of undergraduate students in which many colleges and universities participate to better understand how student learning can be enhanced. The NSSE has established reliability and validity and reflects four themes: (1) *Academic Challenge*, (2) *Learning with Peers*, (3) *Experiences with Faculty*, and (4) *Campus Environment*. Within these themes are a

TABLE 3-1

Engagement Indicators

Theme	Engagement Indicator
Academic Challenge	Higher-Order Learning
	Reflective and Integrative Learning
	Learning Strategies
	Quantitative Reasoning
Learning with Peers	Collaborative Learning
	Discussions with Diverse Others
Experiences with Faculty	Student-Faculty Interaction
	Effective Teaching Practices
Campus Environment	Quality of Interactions
	Supportive Environment

total of 10 engagement Indicators (see Table 3-1) that are separate aspects of engagement identified during psychometric testing of the survey (NSSE, 2015).

The NSSE also identifies six high impact practices that enhance student engagement and learning (see Table 3-2) and recommends that undergraduate students engage in at least two practices during their education with one in the first year and one in their major (NSSE, 2015).

Popkess and McDaniel (2011) and Johnson (2015) reviewed responses to the 2003 NSSE by 1,000 nursing students, 1,000 education majors, and 1,000 other health pre-professional students to gain further insight into nursing student engagement. Nursing students reported a higher level of *Academic Challenge* and working on community projects than other majors; both nursing and health professional majors reported less *Collaborative Learning* than education majors. The authors posited that this latter finding may be related to an underutilization of *Collaborative Learning* activities in nursing and health pre-professional schools at the time.

Johnson (2015) also compared 2003 to 2010 NSSE results from more than 10,000 surveys of undergraduate nursing students as they related specifically to changes in level of *Academic Challenge, Active and Collaborative Learning*, and *Student-Faculty Interaction*. Findings demonstrated small improvements in level of *Academic Challenge* and *Student-Faculty Interactions* over this seven-year time span although this change was considered negligible; in relation to *Active and Collaborative Learning*, there was no change over that same time period. The author recommended enhancing student engagement through a focus on NSSE Indicators, particularly on *Active and Collaborative Learning*.

Docherty et al. (2018) provide an example of how to incorporate NSSE recommendations for student engagement intentionally into the development of pedagogies that address NSSE engagement Indicators. They developed learning activities throughout

TABLE 3-2

High-Impact Practices

Practice	Survey Focus
Service-Learning	Number of courses that have included a community-based project (service-learning)
Learning Community	Participation in a learning community or some other formal program where groups of students take two or more classes together
Research with Faculty	Work with a faculty member on a research project
Internship or Field Experience	Participation in an internship, co-op, field experience, student teaching experience, or clinical placement
Study Abroad	Participation in a study abroad program
Culminating Senior Experience	Completion of a culminating senior experience (capstone course, senior project or thesis, comprehensive exam, portfolio, etc.)

their program of study in a baccalaureate nursing program to meet eight of the ten engagement Indicators, including *Theater of the Oppressed, Simulation as a Clinical Site for Active Engagement, Legal Simulation*, and *Creating Student Researchers.*

In an online environment, student engagement can also be facilitated, although the mechanisms may be different. Linder and Mattison Hayes (2018) provide exemplars of how to design high impact practices for the online environment, including the use of ePortfolios as a way to help students explicate what they have learned across the program of study by reflecting on the various artifacts they produced over time. They note Sparrow and Torok (2018), who assert that ePortfolios also can amplify the effect of other high impact practices such as learning that occurred as a result of internships, global learning experiences, or collaborative projects. Lundberg and Sheridan (2015) evaluated NSSE survey results of 812 undergraduate students enrolled exclusively in online courses and found that the following were the strongest predictors of learning related to general education, personal development, and practical competence: "a supportive campus environment, an institutional emphasis on encouraging contact among students from different backgrounds, and student effort in response to high expectations of faculty" (p. 13).

Because the NSSE specifically looks at undergraduate student engagement, there is a large body of literature identifying best practices in enhancing engagement in this population. However, it is apparent that many of the best practices outlined also support student engagement and enhance learning in graduate education, although supporting literature for graduate populations most commonly comes from majors other than nursing. Reiff and Ballin (2016) collected feedback from 179 graduate students in a hybrid master of education program about positive and negative learning experiences. They identified one theme of engagement from student feedback as contributing to positive learning outcomes. Specifically, students talked about relevant, active learning strategies and faculty creation of a sense of connection within the course as strategies that promoted student engagement. Kuchinski-Donnelly and Krouse (2020) explored the relationship between autonomy, competency, and relatedness (relationships) to emotional engagement in 123 graduate nursing students enrolled in an online master's program. While all three variables of autonomy, competency, and relatedness were positively correlated with emotional engagement, only competency was a significant predictor of such engagement. The authors recommended that faculty be intentional about including competency-building learning activities, such as problem-based assignments, throughout the course to facilitate emotional engagement.

Reflective of evidence such as that described here, the National League for Nursing acknowledges the importance of student engagement to achieve excellence and distinction in nursing education. Specifically, the *Hallmarks of Excellence in Nursing Education©* (2020) in this category identify three areas that faculty should consider as they design curricula and plan approaches to facilitate and evaluate learning:

▸ Students are excited about learning and exhibit a spirit of inquiry as well as a commitment to lifelong learning.

> Students are committed to innovation, continuous quality/performance improvement, and excellence.

> Students are committed to the professional nursing role including advancement in leadership, scholarship, and mentoring.

EXCITEMENT ABOUT LEARNING AND EXHIBITING A SPIRIT OF INQUIRY

In this Hallmark, faculty are encouraged to create learning environments and activities that fully engage both pre-licensure and graduate students, enhance their excitement about learning, encourage their spirit of inquiry, and develop a commitment to lifelong learning. Questions faculty might ask themselves to determine if the program is achieving this Hallmark include the following:

> To what extent do students appraise evidence and use the information discovered to contribute to class and clinical discussions?

> In what ways do students brainstorm together about concepts such as those presented in class and introduced in various references and clinical experiences?

> To what extent do students question if current clinical practices (e.g., approaches to patient care, the way communication occurs on clinical units, existing policies) are based on research and evidence?

> Do students ask "What if" questions?

> In what ways do students demonstrate enthusiasm about continued learning and professional development?

Exemplars discussed in this Hallmark are learning opportunities that facilitate (1) student competency in evidence appraisal and research capacity to improve clinical and nursing knowledge, and (2) collaborative learning techniques that facilitate students working together to improve learning. Creating an academic environment for active nursing student engagement in evidence-based practice (EBP) and research is key to promoting student excitement and interest in continued application of these principles in clinical practice. Understanding facilitators and barriers to implementing such an environment is also of importance. Blackman and Giles (2017), in a descriptive survey of 375 undergraduate nursing students, explored factors associated with students' ability to apply EBP principles. Factors leading to the largest influence on EBP self-efficacy included students' ability to (1) analyze, critique, and synthesize existing research; (2) apply the mechanics of research; and (3) communicate research results to staff and patients. In a scoping review of 37 research studies on undergraduate nursing student use of EBP (Fiset et al., 2017), one aspect was to identify barriers that influence student practices, the most often reported ones being lack of knowledge and negative attitudes about EBP. Educational strategies had the largest influence on improving knowledge and attitudes in the studies reviewed. Recommendations from both Blackman and Giles (2017) and Fiset et al. (2017) include situating undergraduate EBP education in classroom instruction as well as in clinical application focusing on utilizing information literacy and research knowledge to apply to authentic clinical problems and questions (Aglen, 2016). This recommendation would seem applicable for graduate education as well.

Several faculty groups have taken an integrated curricular approach to design EBP and/or research learning activities that provide multiple opportunities for student engagement with EBP and/or research activities, including dissemination, throughout the program of study. Ross et al. (2009) described a curricular approach of seven learning activities embedded throughout a three-year undergraduate curriculum that applied knowledge development of EBP principles through case study and simulated scenarios, and then through clinical application culminating in a clinical outcomes project. Ayoola et al. (2017) designed a systems approach at another undergraduate program with multiple opportunities to engage with research, including knowledge development in the classroom, faculty mentoring, and clinical application through community assessments. Students also had the opportunity to participate in a university-wide honors program, and faculty advisement included consideration of doctoral education. Docherty et al. (2018), in their design of learning activities to align with NSSE recommendations for undergraduate student engagement, also utilized faculty mentoring as well as collaborative student learning to facilitate engagement with research and EBP. They identified that the strategy of *Creating Student Researchers* employed the NSSE engagement Indicators of *Collaborative Learning*, *Effective Teaching Practices*, *Quality of Interactions*, and *Supportive Environment*.

While virtually all doctoral nursing students engage in inquiry related to translational science or knowledge development, the opportunity to participate in research and EBP initiatives may be more variable in master's students. O'Connor et al. (2016) describe an initiative in which master's level students participated in an interdisciplinary research study on aging in rural areas by recruiting subjects, collecting data, and disseminating findings. They concluded that providing master's level students with an opportunity to participate in faculty research can facilitate engagement and professional development.

Collaborative Learning is an NSSE engagement Indicator and includes opportunities for students to learn as a team, perhaps through problem-based learning, and engage in peer assessment. Stone et al. (2013) performed a systematic review of 18 studies to evaluate the benefits of peer learning to undergraduate nursing students. The studies reviewed included a variety of peer learning techniques, such as peer tutoring, coaching, and problem-based learning. Sixteen of the studies demonstrated benefits to students including increases in student satisfaction, confidence, and critical thinking skills as well as a decrease in anxiety. Problem-based learning supported theoretical learning primarily while other forms of collaborative learning such as role-play, peer mentoring, and coaching benefited both theoretical and clinical learning.

An increase in student engagement was demonstrated in several other studies that examined collaborative or team-based learning in both undergraduate and graduate students. One study reported that undergraduate political science students were more active in the class (Hermann, 2013), and another study reported higher levels of peer interactions in postgraduate critical care nursing students (Currey et al., 2015). Mennenga (2013) compared a team-based learning strategy with traditional classroom lecture in a study of 143 undergraduate nursing students in a community health course. The team-based learning strategy included pre-class preparation and then, in class, individual testing followed by group testing with immediate feedback and discussion of concepts. While testing performance was unchanged, students in the team-based learning section reported higher levels of engagement.

Nichols et al. (2016) describe the positive benefits of team-based learning that can occur in graduate nursing online learning environments. In this study, learning teams of three students each complete all aspects of the course assignments as a team. Evaluations from students and faculty were overwhelmingly positive with students reporting improved critical thinking, peer support, and feedback, while faculty identified improved social and teaching presence, both of which are factors in student engagement.

In the online environment, adopting an evidence-based framework, such as the Community of Inquiry Model, can facilitate student engagement through intentional design and attention to cognitive, social, and teaching presences within a course to support meaningful education experiences and student interaction (Fiock, 2020). *Cognitive presence* refers to the ability of learners to construct meaning through interaction with course content and others in the course through collaborative inquiry, discussion, and reflection. *Social presence* refers to the ability to express oneself emotionally, communicate with others, feel part of a group of learners, and perceive self and others in the course as real people. *Teaching presence* refers to the support of meaningful learning through course design, facilitation of discussion, and direct instruction. A structural equation model study by Kucuk and Ricardson (2019) of 123 graduate students in online courses demonstrated that cognitive, social, and teaching presences have positive effects on student engagement in graduate courses; interestingly, teaching presence was found to be the strongest predictor of student satisfaction.

In a multicampus survey of student engagement of 186 students across multiple online courses, Dixson (2010) described a higher level of engagement by students who reported they interacted with peers and the teacher in multiple ways. This researcher recommended that assignments be constructed in ways that facilitate student interaction with the faculty member, the content, and each other in an effort to enhance social, cognitive, and teaching presences. Fiock (2020) summarizes a myriad of online activities that support the Community of Inquiry Model and promote teaching presence: timely feedback on assignments and faculty engagement in forum discussions; enhancing social presence by creating an introduction forum for learners and faculty to introduce themselves and short faculty videos introducing self or topics; and using grading rubrics, peer review, and reflection to enhance cognitive presence.

In summary, thoughtfully designed learning activities to engage students with authentic clinical application of research and EBP can fulfill many aspects of this Hallmark. Crafting learning activities to ensure knowledge and skill development in information literacy and appraisal of evidence along with collaborative approaches to clinically based inquiry are key to engage students in becoming and staying excited throughout their career in problem solving to improve practice. Research with faculty, internships or field experiences, and culminating senior experiences all are identified by the NSSE as high impact practices for student engagement. Clinically based EBP projects promote student engagement and are naturally aligned with internships or field experiences as well as with culminating senior experiences (NSSE, 2015). *Collaborative Learning* also is an engagement Indicator in NSSE that facilitates student engagement through *Learning with Peers* and *Interacting with Faculty*.

COMMITMENT TO INNOVATION, CONTINUOUS IMPROVEMENT, AND EXCELLENCE

In order to help students understand the importance of this Hallmark that addresses innovation and continuous quality/performance improvement and excellence, as well as to encourage and support their ongoing commitment to each, faculty can reflect on the extent to which the following Indicators of this Hallmark are evident in their academic programs:

> To what extent do students respond to critical/constructive feedback and then use that feedback to make improvements in their performance?

> In what ways are students open to trying new things?

> In what ways are students stimulated in their learning when innovative teaching strategies are integrated into the classroom, lab, and/or clinical setting?

> In what ways do students reflect on their own performance and experiences in order to be proactive in implementing improved performance?

> In what ways do students observe for areas of quality improvement within systems and suggest appropriate solutions?

> In what ways are students incorporating technology to make improvements in their performance?

This Hallmark can be achieved through the use of learning strategies that are innovative, use technology effectively, challenge students to be reflective and insightful about themselves and their performance, encourage students to attend to "the big picture," and effectively integrate classroom, lab, and clinical learning. Exemplars of activities that reflect these ideas and can close the theory practice gap include global travel and service learning – both of which are considered NSSE high-impact practices – as well as simulation, which is an example of the engagement Indicator of *Reflective and Integrative Learning*. Other strategies that enhance student engagement include reflection and peer assessment – both of which align with the NSSE engagement Indicators of *Reflective and Integrative Learning* and *Collaborative Learning* – in which internal and external feedback are used to improve performance and enhance self-understanding. Innovative learning strategies can stimulate students through multiple engagement Indicators in the thematic areas of *Academic Challenge*, *Learning with Peers*, and *Interactions with Faculty*.

Indicators of the Hallmark related to innovation, continuous improvement, and excellence are supported by findings that identify learning activities nursing faculty intentionally select to engage students. For example, one literature review and thematic analysis of findings in undergraduate nursing studies (Crookes et al., 2013) identified the following subsets of learning activities that faculty intentionally use to engage students: reflection, simulation, online learning, gaming, art, problem/context-based learning, and narrative teaching techniques. Reflection is an oral or written focused review and evaluation of a recent experience in order to improve performance or to link it to past experiences to make connections and deepen learning (Brown et al., 2014; Crookes et al., 2013). Such an activity has multiple learner benefits in that it can strengthen the

connection between theory and practice and cement long-term learning through information retrieval practices that facilitate critical thinking and clinical judgment (Brown
et al., 2014; Crookes et al., 2013).

Henderson et al. (2018) describe a consistent process called Check In – Check Out
(CICO) used across undergraduate laboratory, simulation, and clinical learning settings
that incorporates reflection at both checkpoints. Immediately before clinical learning
activities, the student answers a series of four questions:

> What will I be doing today? This answer helps to confirm alignment of student and
> faculty expectations.

> What questions do I have before starting? This response provides an opportunity
> for the student to seek clarification.

> What are my learning goals? This answer makes explicit student-specific learning
> goals.

> What am I learning about today? This response provides the student an opportunity
> to consider all areas for potential learning related to patient-centered, safe, and
> evidence-based care.

These questions aid in making explicit what the student does and does not know. At
Check Out, there is a debriefing reflection to evaluate and improve performance. Evaluation of this process by students and faculty revealed CICO to be an effective student
engagement practice.

Another strategy to enhance self-reflection and performance improvement is reflective clinical journaling (Lasater & Nielsen, 2009), a process that aligns with Tanner's clinical judgment model (Tanner, 2006) and addresses the following aspects: background,
noticing, interpreting, responding, and reflecting. The study conducted by Lasater and
Nielsen revealed that this process helped to illustrate student thinking and clinical judgment and provided an opportunity to strengthen learning by uncovering and correcting
faulty thinking.

In addition to these reflective practices, *Collaborative Learning* also facilitates student engagement and performance improvement, particularly through seeking feedback
from and providing feedback to peers. Casey et al. (2011) evaluated the impact of peer
assessment on student engagement and found that the 37 undergraduate students who
provided feedback on two assignments completed by peers reported that engaging in
peer assessment improved their own learning, helped them better understand the assignment, and helped them improve their own performance. Findings of an integrative
review of 24 studies in undergraduate and graduate nursing education on peer assessment conducted by Tornwall (2018) revealed that peer assessment and feedback (1) is
used across classroom, laboratory, and clinical learning settings; (2) supports student
engagement, critical thinking, and improved self-assessment and performance; and
(3) is most effective when used in a trusting environment and when students are prepared to conduct peer assessments through practice opportunities and exemplars.

Another strategy – the use of technology, particularly gaming or virtual communities,
whether in online or face-to-face environments – also can engage students, especially
digital natives, due to the interactive nature of games and the ability to connect theory
with practice (Crookes et al., 2013). A classroom response system (CRS) is one type

of gaming that has evolved from hand-held clickers to online polling through smartphones or computers. This gaming method is primarily used for formative assessment and has been found to contribute to student engagement, assist both students and faculty to identify gaps in understanding, and promote information retrieval practices to cement long-term learning (De Gagne, 2011). In a seminal research study, Berry (2009) evaluated the introduction of hand-held clickers into the classroom and identified improvements in final grades, student engagement, and satisfaction. The importance of CRSs to formative assessment were supported by Sheng et al. (2019) in a study of the benefits of CRSs to students enrolled in both traditional and accelerated undergraduate programs, which demonstrated improved learning and participation. De Gagne (2011) recommended that CRSs are best incorporated with faculty clarification of concepts to address gaps in understanding. Faculty can identify areas for further explanation and teaching based on incorrect class responses.

Virtual communities, another type of technology innovation, also contribute to student engagement. Virtual communities are web-based simulated neighborhoods in which students learn about health issues or other professional topics by engaging in a contextualized environment where stories of individuals, families, and communities unfold over time, and faculty facilitate discussion of how those stories relate to course outcomes. Findings from a study of undergraduate students enrolled in a course that used a virtual community compared to the same course that used traditional learning activities revealed greater learner engagement in the course with the virtual community (Giddens et al., 2012).

Service learning, whether global or local, also can provide innovative opportunities for student engagement that allows for integration of theory with practice, as well as experiences with system assessment and improvement. Service learning connects theory with practice through civic engagement and provides benefits to the learners and to the community organization served. Dombrowsky et al. (2019) examined nurse educators' understanding of the similarities and differences between service learning and the clinical learning experiences that are typical in nursing education programs. These researchers found that nurse educators were confused regarding the terms and highlighted the need to differentiate the two and clarify that not all clinical education is service learning. In essence, service learning is driven primarily by a desire to meet a community need while clinical education is driven by a desire to help students learn the practice of nursing.

One additional strategy – study abroad experiences – has been shown to be successful in engaging students and helping them better understand global health and the nursing profession across different international settings. Kulbok et al. (2012) performed a literature review of 23 studies of study abroad in undergraduate and graduate programs and identified that most programs are instituted to provide students opportunities to enhance their understandings of diverse populations. Dohrn et al. (2018) describe an ongoing global learning experience available to master's and doctoral students enrolled in accelerated programs in which students describe an increased understanding of health disparities and how nursing practice differs in countries with varying resources.

Both service learning and study abroad experiences can be situated within the program of study or in extracurricular activities through student service or other organizations. Rodriguez and Lapiz-Bluhm (2018) interviewed 12 undergraduate nursing students who completed an extracurricular health screening service learning project in their local community; those students reported multiple benefits including the opportunity to give back to the community, a feeling of being engaged with the community, and a sense of empowerment, which helped them better understand systems and system improvement. DeBonis (2016) describes a service-learning opportunity for graduate nursing students in nurse practitioner and nursing education tracts through a free nurse-run clinic that the university established with the local Salvation Army. In a study of 152 graduate nurse students who experienced this service-learning opportunity that focused on providing preventative care and education, there was a significant increase post-experience in students' civic engagement, as evidenced by their desire to volunteer in their community, as well as an increase in cultural competency and knowledge of underserved populations.

Service-learning can be combined with other teaching techniques to enhance student engagement. Noone et al. (2019) describe an undergraduate study abroad serving-learning experience that is combined with pre- and post-experience reflection to maximize student engagement. Faculty in the host community work with community agencies to design service-learning experiences for visiting students. Students work with the local community agencies to complete community assessments in their host community and have an opportunity to learn about nursing and health care in a different country. Shannon (2019) describes a multiterm service-learning experience involving multiple cohorts of students to promote community disaster preparedness as well as multiple methods for student engagement such as reflection and gaming. Waldner et al. (2012) described the types of e-service-learning possible in which all or part of the instruction and/or service occur online, and they recommend best practices for technology, communication, and course design that are essential to support such an approach. Assessment and training of the technological capacity of the community partner as well as engagement of the community partner in participating in the course within the learning management system are identified best practices for e-service-learning. Exemplars of e-service-learning that relate to nursing include online mentoring programs and the development of websites and online community interest and advocacy groups. Other examples included audits of policies and procedures or community assessments that were conducted virtually and communicated to community partners through the course management system or via videoconferencing systems.

In summary, the structure of nursing education as professionally grounded and clinically based is well-situated to evolve meaningful activities that enhance students' commitment to innovation, continuous improvement, and excellence that align with this Hallmark. Further integration of reflection into student self-evaluation can enhance student engagement in their own progression. Many clinical learning activities may be able to be adapted to service-learning activities or expanded to include global learning. Innovative teaching strategies in the classroom setting can further close the theory-practice gap, facilitate student engagement in learning, and enhance students' development as clinicians, leaders, and scholars.

COMMITMENT TO A PROFESSIONAL NURSING ROLE: LEADERSHIP, SCHOLARSHIP, AND MENTORING

One final aspect of the importance of fully engaging students in the learning process in order to achieve excellence in nursing education relates to their commitment to the professional nursing role. In addition to the role involving care delivery, excellence is achieved when students also develop an identity as leaders, scholars, and mentors, and determining the extent to which this goal has been achieved can be assessed by responses to the following questions:

> In what ways do students express anticipatory excitement about professional identity formation, continuing their education, pursuing graduate study, assuming leadership roles in their employment settings and in the profession, serving as mentors, and becoming actively involved in professional associations? How do they express excitement about the contributions they hope to make to the nursing profession?

> In what ways do students propose a realistic short- and long-term career trajectory for themselves?

> To what extent do students collaborate with others to create environments that are civil, inclusive, respectful, and promote excellence?

> In what ways do students provide evidence of seeing themselves as being responsible for advancing the profession of nursing?

Professional identity formation and collaborative professional behavior development are key aspects of this Hallmark and can be facilitated through the NSSE engagement Indicator of *Faculty-Student Interactions*, through which faculty can be role models, mentors, or advisors as students transition to practice. Additionally, effective academic-clinical partnerships, involvement in professional nursing organizations, and other activities can help to close the theory-practice gap, facilitate successful transition to practice, promote professional development, and foster collaboration, respect, and civility. The intentional design of learning activities throughout the program, but particularly toward its end, can facilitate successful transition to practice as students look forward to graduation, employment, or graduate school.

Meyer et al. (2017) reported increased job satisfaction at the three-month employment mark for students who participated in a revised curriculum focused on transition to practice. The revised curriculum included theoretical knowledge development and simulation learning activities related to practice safety issues such as near misses and lateral violence, as well as career development activities such as interview practice and resume writing. Church et al. (2019) developed a transition-to-practice toolkit to assist learners to evaluate components of a healthy work environment as they seek employment. This toolkit and set of activities align with the American Nurses Credentialing Center (ANCC) Practice Transition Accreditation Program™ (PTAP™) Conceptual Model (ANCC, n.d.).

Clinical and community partners may be excellent resources to facilitate transition to practice and professional formation. Martin (2016) describes a faculty-student toolkit that a state nursing association developed to assist student connection with their professional nursing organization and includes transition-to-practice activities such as preparation for employment and practice. Career planning, mentoring, and transition-to-practice workshops were described by Noone et al. (2020) and included a Graduate Exploration Workshop to explore graduate school as part of student career planning. In addition, students completed a career plan with their mentor. A triad mentoring project that involved the student, faculty, and a practice partner was described by Dolan and Willson (2019) for graduate students in a master's program in Leadership and Nursing Administration, which facilitated transition to the practice world and could be adapted for undergraduate students.

There has been a recent emphasis on civility in nursing for both practicing nurses and students to reduce workplace and lateral violence. Strategies to engage students in developing professional behaviors, including civility and respect, can foster teamwork and collaboration that can carry over into professional nursing practice. Clark (2017) outlines several strategies that programs can use to frame professional behaviors and integrate learning these professional behaviors throughout the curriculum. For example, setting the stage for a framework of the expectation of civility within the academic environment can be enhanced by having a civility statement within the program of study as well as offering a "White Coat" ceremony for new students that welcomes students into the profession and provides an opportunity for them to publicly commit to professional practice. Embedding active learning strategies throughout the curriculum focused on the development of civil and respectful behaviors was also a recommended strategy. Clark and Dunham (2020) describe a series of virtual learning activities, called the "Civility Mentor," that provides foundational knowledge as students enter the program and incorporates additional learning activities that apply to the academic and clinical environments as students progress through the program of study and transition to practice. Students reported that the "Civility Mentor" was effective in providing them with strategies to approach incivility and improve communication. Parker and McMillan (2020) describe the use of an e-Portfolio with master's in nursing education students to focus awareness on development of skills in communication, teamwork, and civility. These authors posited the importance of this self-awareness in graduate students who will become the leaders in nursing academic and practice settings.

In summary, partnerships with community and professional organizations can facilitate student transition to practice. Intentional design of learning activities to enhance professional identity formation and behaviors, such as respect, collaboration, and civility, is critical to student commitment to the professional role.

CONCLUSION

There is a growing body of nursing education literature regarding strategies that can enhance the engagement of students in the educational process and thereby facilitate their academic and career success. As previously noted, there are many opportunities within the program of study to revise learning activities to meet the Hallmarks outlined in this chapter and improve student engagement. In conclusion, some recommendations to consider for improving student engagement are outlined in the following list:

> Align the curriculum with evidence-based models such as the engagement Indicators and high-impact practices identified by the NSSE or through adoption of a Community of Inquiry framework for online programs. Several nursing programs discussed how they implemented a framework to engage students that was either embedded in several courses (Docherty et al., 2018; Meyer et al., 2017) or throughout the curriculum (Henderson et al., 2018). Consider adopting the recommendation of incorporating at least two high impact practices in the program of study (NSSE, 2015). Popkess and McDaniel (2011) and Johnson (2015), in their reviews of undergraduate nursing students' responses on the NSSE, recommended enhancing opportunities in nursing education for collaborative learning.

> When designing innovative teaching classroom and clinical learning activities, the importance of effective instructional design cannot be overemphasized. It is imperative to provide foundational knowledge to prepare learners for academic success. For example, supporting students with foundational knowledge about how to be an effective peer reviewer would facilitate student success when implementing peer review strategies. Provide consistent faculty contact and follow-up to clarify concepts and correct gaps in knowledge when using interactive learning strategies. Faculty development and mentoring for effective instructional design of high impact practices is critical to implement and understand nontraditional teaching methods, such as online teaching or service learning (McNair & Albertine, 2012).

> Academic-practice partnerships that link classroom learning to authentic clinical application were identified as a strategy for all three of the Hallmarks addressed in this chapter. In addition to providing traditional clinical learning experiences, such partnerships can facilitate student engagement with authentic EBP projects, provide opportunities for service learning, and optimize transition to practice.

> Several exemplars discussed combining multiple student engagement techniques into a learning activity, such as using reflection in a service learning or global experience. Learning activities could also integrate techniques across these three Hallmarks, such as developing an evidence-based project related to professional role development. The cumulative impact of incorporating multiple high impact practices has been supported by an analysis of NSSE surveys of 25,336 students at 38 institutions in California, Oregon, and Wisconsin (Finley & McNair, 2013). This analysis revealed that participating in multiple high impact practices had a cumulative effect with students reporting higher gains in learning and personal and social development.

> The importance of *Student-Faculty Interactions* as an engagement Indicator is vital for faculty to recognize and intentionally incorporate throughout the curriculum. In addition to acting as role models and mentors, faculty can stimulate student interest in research and career planning.

> The nursing education literature provides substantial evidence-based teaching strategies focused on student engagement, especially supported through original research or evaluating a body of research through scoping or systematic reviews. Consider evaluating outcomes of innovations developed and adding to the body of knowledge regarding methods to enhance nursing student engagement.

Whatever the strategy or approach used, designing curricula and selecting strategies to facilitate and evaluate student engagement in the learning process is critical. It is clear that such engagement can be achieved when faculty challenge themselves to be innovative, evidence-based, and student-centered; and the outcomes of such efforts are very worthwhile.

References

Aglen, B. (2016). Pedagogical strategies to teach bachelor students evidence-based practice: A systematic review. *Nurse Education Today, 36*, 255–263. https://doi.org/10.1016/j.nedt.2015.08.025

American Nurses Credentialing Center. (n.d.). *Practice transition accreditation program (PTAP).* https://www.nursingworld.org/organizational-programs/accreditation/ptap/

Ayoola, A. B., Adams, Y. J., Kamp, K. J., Zandee, G. L., Feenstra, C., & Doornbos, M. M. (2017). Promoting the future of nursing by increasing zest for research in undergraduate nursing students. *Journal of Professional Nursing, 33*(2), 126–132. https://doi.org/10.1016/j.profnurs.2016.08.011

Bernard, J. S. (2015). Student engagement: A principle-based concept analysis. *International Journal of Nursing Education Scholarship, 12*(1), 1–11. https://doi.org/10.1515/ijnes-2014-0058

Berry, J. (2009). Technology support in nursing education: Clickers in the classroom. *Nursing Education Perspectives, 30*(5), 295–298.

Blackman, I. R., & Giles, T. M. (2017). Can nursing students practice what is preached? Factors impacting graduating nurses' abilities and achievement to apply evidence-based practices. *Worldviews on Evidence-Based Nursing, 14*(2), 108–117. https://doi.org/10.1111/wvn.12205

Bowcock, R., & Peters, K. (2016). Discussion paper: Conceptual comparison of student and therapeutic engagement. *Nurse Education in Practice, 17*, 188–191. https://doi.org/10.1016/j.nepr.2015.10.010

Brown, P. C., Roediger III., H. L., & McDaniel, M. A. (2014). *Make it stick: The science of successful learning.* Harvard University Press.

Casey, D., Burke, E., Houghton, C., Mee, L., Smith, R., Van Der Putten, D., Bradley, H., & Folan, M. (2011). Use of peer assessment as a student engagement strategy in nurse education. *Nursing & Health Sciences, 13*(4), 514–520. https://doi.org/10.1111/j.1442-2018.2011.00637.x

Church, C. D., White, M., & Cosme, S. (2019). Helping students identify a healthy transition-to-practice work environment. *Nurse Educator, 45*(4), 174–176. https://doi.org/10.1097/NNE.0000000000000751

Clark, C. M. (2017). An evidence-based approach to integrate civility, professionalism, and ethical practice into nursing curricula. *Nurse Educator, 42*(3), 120–126. https://doi.org/10.1097/NNE.0000000000000331

Clark, C. M., & Dunham, M. (2020). Civility mentor: A virtual learning experience. *Nurse Educator, 45*(4), 189–192. https://doi.org/10.1097/NNE.0000000000000757

Crookes, K., Crookes, P. A., & Walsh, K. (2013). Meaningful and engaging teaching techniques for student nurses: A literature review. *Nurse Education in Practice, 13*(4), 239–243. https://doi.org/10.1016/j.nepr.2013.04.008

Currey, J., Oldland, E., Considine, J., Glanville, D., & Story, I. (2015). Evaluation of postgraduate critical care nursing students' attitudes to, and engagement with, team-based learning: A descriptive study. *Intensive & Critical Care Nursing, 31*(1), 19–28. https://doi.org/10.1016/j.iccn.2014.09.003

DeBonis, R. (2016). Effects of service-learning on graduate nursing students: Care and advocacy for the impoverished. *Journal of Nursing Education, 55*(1), 36–40. https://doi.org/10.3928/01484834-20151214-09

De Gagne, J. C. (2011). The impact of clickers in nursing education: A review of literature. *Nurse Education Today, 31*(8), e34–e40. https://doi.org/10.1016/j.nedt.2010.12.007

Dixson, M. D. (2010). Creating effective student engagement in online courses: What do students find engaging? *Journal of the Scholarship of Teaching and Learning, 10*(2). 1–13.

Docherty, A., Warkentin, P., Borgen, J., Garthe, K. A., Fischer, K. L, & Halabi Najjara, R. (2018). Enhancing student engagement: Innovative strategies for intentional learning. *Journal of Professional Nursing, 34*(6), 470–474. https://doi.org/10.1016/j.profnurs.2018.05.001

Dohrn, J., Desjardins, K., Honig, J., Hahn-Schroeder, H., Ferng, Y., & Larson, E. (2018). Transforming nursing curricula for a global community. *Journal of Professional Nursing, 34*(6), 449–453. https://doi.org/10.1016/j.profnurs.2018.02.001

Dolan, D. M., & Willson, P. (2019). Triad mentoring model: Framing an academic–clinical partnership practicum. *Journal of Nursing Education, 58*(8), 463–467. https://doi.org/10.3928/01484834-20190719-05

Dombrowsky, T., Gustafson, K., & Cauble, D. (2019). Service-learning and clinical nursing education: A Delphi inquiry. *Journal of Nursing Education, 58*(7), 381–391. https://doi.org/10.3928/01484834-20190614-02

Finley, A., & McNair, T. (2013). *Assessing underserved students' engagement in high-impact practices.* Association of American Colleges and Universities.

Fiock, H. S. (2020). Designing a Community of Inquiry in online courses. *International Review of Research in Open and Distributed Learning, 21*(1), 135–153. https://doi.org/10.19173/irrodl.v20i5.3985

Fiset, V. J., Graham, I. D., & Davies, B. L. (2017). Evidence-based practice in clinical nursing education: A scoping review. *Journal of Nursing Education, 56*(9), 534–541. https://Ýoi.org/10.3928/01484834-20170817-04

Giddens, J., Hrabe, D., Carlson-Sabelli, L., Fogg, L., & North, S. (2012). The impact of a virtual community on student engagement and academic performance among baccalaureate nursing students. *Journal of Professional Nursing, 28*(5), 284–290. https://doi.org/10.1016/j.profnurs.2012.04.011

Harper, S. R., & Quaye, S. J. (2015). Making engagement equitable for students in U.S. higher education. In S. J. Quaye & S. R. Harper (Eds.), *Student engagement in higher education theoretical perspectives and practical approaches for diverse populations* (2nd ed., pp. 1–14). Routledge.

Henderson, A., Harrison, P., Rowe, J., Edwards, S., Barnes, M., & Henderson, S. (2018). Students take the lead for learning in practice: A process for building self-efficacy into undergraduate nursing education. *Nurse Education in Practice, 31*, 14–19. https://doi.org./10.1016/j.nepr.2018.04.003

Hermann, K. J. (2013). The impact of cooperative learning on student engagement: Results from an intervention. *Active Learning in Higher Education, 14*(3) 175–187. https://doi.org/10.1177/1469787413498035

Hudson, K., & Carrasco, R. (2015). Researching nursing students' engagement: Successful findings for nursing. *International Journal of Nursing & Clinical Practices, 2*(1), 1–5. https://doi.org/10.15344/2394-4978/2015/150

Johnson, K. Z. (2015). *Student engagement in nursing school: A secondary analysis of the National Survey of Student Engagement data.* [Unpublished doctoral dissertation]. Retrieved from University of Kansas: kuscholarworks.ku.edu/bitstream/handle/1808/19449/Johnson_ku_0099D_14023_DATA_1.pdf

Kuchinski-Donnelly, D., & Krouse, A. M. (2020). Predictors of emotional engagement in online graduate nursing students. *Nurse Educator, 45*(4), 214–219. https://doi.org/10.1097/NNE.0000000000000769

Kucuk, S., & Richardson, J. C. (2019). A structural equation model of predictors of online learners' engagement and satisfaction.

Online Learning, 23(2), 196–216. https://doi
.org/10.24059/olj.v23i2.1455

Kulbok, P. A., Mitchell, E. M., Glick, D. F., &
Greiner, D. (2012). International experiences
in nursing education: A review of the
literature. *International Journal of Nursing
Education Scholarship, 9*, 1–21. https://doi
.org/10.1515/1548-923X.2365

Lasater, K., & Nielsen, A. (2009). Reflective
journaling for clinical judgment development
and evaluation. *Journal of Nursing
Education, 48*(1), 40–44. https://doi
.org/10.3928/01484834-20090101-06

Linder, K. E., & Mattison Hayes, C. (Eds.).
(2018). High-impact practices in online
education. *Stylus.*

Lundberg, C. A., & Sheridan, D. (2015).
Benefits of engagement with peers, faculty,
and diversity for online learners. *College
Teaching, 63*, 8–15. https://doi.org/10.1080/
87567555.2014.972317

Martin, E. (2016). District activity: Faculty &
student engagement toolkit. *Texas Nursing,
90*(3), 9.

McNair, T., & Albertine, S. (2012). *Seeking
high-quality, high-impact learning: The
imperative of faculty development and
curricular intentionality.* Association of
American Colleges and Universities.

Mennenga, H. A. (2013). Student engagement
and examination performance in a team-
based learning course. *Journal of Nursing
Education, 52*(8), 475–479. https://doi
.org/10.3928/01484834-20130718-04

Meyer, G., Shatto, B., Delicath, T., &
von der Lancken, S. (2017). Effect
of curriculum revision on graduates'
transition to practice. *Nurse Educator,
42*(3), 127–132. https://doi.org/10.1097/
NNE.0000000000000325

National League for Nursing. (2020). *Hallmarks
of excellence in nursing education.*
http://www.nln.org/docs/default-source/
default-document-library/hallmarks_of_
excellence_2019.pdf?sfvrsn=0

National Survey of Student Engagement.
(2015). *Engagement Indicators & high-
impact practices.* https://www.udmercy.edu/
academics/special/ honors/images/High-
Impact-Practices.pdf

Nichols, M. R., Malone, A., & Esden, J. (2016).
Learning teams and the online learner.
Nurse Educator, 41(2), 62–63. https://doi
.org/10.1097/NNE.0000000000000209

Noone, J., Kohan, T., Hernandez, M. T.,
Tibbetts, D., & Richmond, R. (2019).
Fostering global health practice:
An undergraduate nursing student
exchange and international service-learning
program. *Journal of Nursing Education,
58*(4), 235–239. https://doi.org/
10.3928/01484834-20190321-09

Noone, J., Najjar, R., Koithan, M. S., Quintana,
A. D., & Vaughn, S. (2020). Nursing
workforce diversity: Promising educational
practices. *Journal of Professional Nursing,
36*(5), 386–394. https://doi.org/10.1016/j
.profnurs.2020.02.011

O'Connor, M. L., Fuller-Iglesias, H., Bishop,
A. J., Doll, G., Killian, T., Margrett, J.,
& Pearson-Scott, J. (2016). Engaging
graduate-level distance learners in research:
A collaborative investigation of rural aging.
Gerontology & Geriatrics Education, 37(1),
29–42. https://doi.org/10.1080/02701960
.2015.1127808

Parker, F. M., & McMillan, L. R. (2020). Using
e-Portfolio to showcase and enhance soft
skill reflection of MSN students. *Journal of
Nursing Education, 59*(5), 300. https://doi
.org/10.3928/01484834-20200422-16

Popkess, A. M., & McDaniel, D. (2011). Are
nursing students engaged in learning? A
secondary analysis of data from the national
survey of student engagement. *Nursing
Education Perspectives, 32*(2), 89–94.
https://doi.org/10.5480/1536-5026-32.2.89

Reiff, M., & Ballin, A. (2016). Adult graduate
student voices: Good and bad learning
experiences. *Adult Learning, 27*(2), 76–83.
https://doi.org/10.1177/1045159516629927

Rodriguez, Y., & Lapiz-Bluhm, M. D.
(2018). Community service learning in
undergraduate nursing: Impact and insights
among students. *Journal of Nursing Practice
Applications & Reviews of Research,
8*(2), 42–49. https://doi.org/10.13178/
jnparr.2018.0802.0807

Ross, A. M., Noone, J., Luce, L., & Sideras, S.
(2009). Spiraling evidence-based practice

and outcomes management concepts in an undergraduate curriculum: A systematic approach. *Journal of Nursing Education, 48*(6), 319–326. https://doi.org/10.3928/01484834-20090515-04

Shannon, C. (2019). Improving student engagement in community disaster preparedness. *Nurse Educator, 44*(6), 304–307. https://doi.org/10.1097/NNE.0000000000000645

Sheng, R., Goldie, C. L., Pulling, C., & Luctkar-Flude, M. (2019). Evaluating student perceptions of a multi-platform classroom response system in undergraduate nursing. *Nurse Education Today, 78*, 25–31. https://doi.org/10.1016/j.nedt.2019.03.008

Sparrow, J., & Torok, J. (2018). ePortfolios. In K. E. Linder & C. Mattison Hayes (Eds.), *High-impact practices in online education* (pp. 183–195). Stylus.

Stone, R., Cooper, S., & Cant, R. (2013). The value of peer learning in undergraduate nursing education: A systematic review.

ISRN Nursing, 2013, 1–10. https://doi.org/10.1155/2013/930901

Tanner, C. A. (2006). Thinking like a nurse: A research-based model of clinical judgment in nursing. *Journal of Nursing Education, 45*(6), 204–211. https://doi.org/10.3928/01484834-20060601-04

Tornwall, J. (2018). Peer assessment practices in nurse education: An integrative review. *Nurse Education Today, 71*, 266–275. https://doi.org/10.1016/j.nedt.2018.09.017

Waldner, L. S., McGorry, S. Y., & Widener, M. C. (2012). E-service-learning: The evolution of service-learning to engage a growing online student population. *Journal of Higher Education Outreach and Engagement, 16*(2), 123–149.

Xerri, M. J., Radford, K., & Shacklock, K. (2018). Student engagement in academic activities: A social support perspective. *Higher Education, 75*(4), 589–605. https://doi.org/10.1007/s10734-017-0162-9

4

Diverse, Well-Prepared Faculty: Essential to Ensuring Excellence and Achieving Distinction in Nursing Education

Jacquelyn McMillian-Bohler, PhD, CNM, CNE

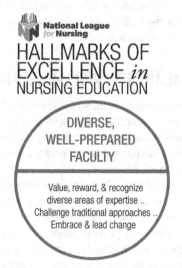

National League for Nursing

HALLMARKS OF EXCELLENCE *in* NURSING EDUCATION

DIVERSE, WELL-PREPARED FACULTY

Value, reward, & recognize diverse areas of expertise ..
Challenge traditional approaches ..
Embrace & lead change

INTRODUCTION

Excellence in nursing education is inextricably linked to the quality of the faculty who are responsible for all aspects of nursing curriculum and program evaluation. In addition to direct instruction and mentorship, faculty contribute to practice and educational standards through research and scholarship, and influence nursing practice and education through community engagement and involvement in professional organizations. To achieve distinction and excellence in nursing education, given the broad influence of nursing faculty, they must be well-prepared for the role.

Expertise in a clinical, leadership, or research setting does not automatically prepare a nurse to achieve excellence as an educator (Booth et al., 2016). Nurse educators are responsible for assisting learners from diverse backgrounds and experiences to acquire and then apply complex knowledge in practice. Knowing *what* to teach and knowing *how* to teach are distinctly different skill sets (Valiga, 2017). Understanding how to engage students and support individual learning needs requires a distinct type of expertise (Booth et al., 2016). Ensuring there is a diverse body of well-prepared nurse educators requires clear guidelines, standards, and planning.

Since the first edition of this book in 2009, publications outlining criteria for nurse educators have been issued or updated, including the National League for Nursing (NLN) Core Competencies for Nurse Educators: A Decade of Influence (Halstead, 2018), *Core Competencies*, the NLN Scope of Practice for Nurse Educators and Academic Clinical Nurse Educators (Christensen & Simmons, 2019), *Teaching in Nursing* (Billings & Halstead, 2019), the *NLN Program Outcomes and Competencies for Graduate Academic Nurse Educator Preparation* (NLN, 2017), and the World Health Organization (WHO) *Nurse Educator Competencies* (2016). Being "well-prepared" implies an elevated level of preparedness, and faculty may need guidance in determining what is required to achieve this type of distinction. This chapter discusses the need to prepare diverse faculty for the complexity of the educator role, so they have the knowledge, skills, and confidence to design, implement, and evaluate academic programs that represent excellence and distinction in nursing education.

DEFINING WHAT IS MEANT BY "WELL-PREPARED FACULTY"

The NLN's Hallmarks of Excellence in Nursing Education© (NLN, 2020), along with the Indicators for each, outline the characteristics of well-prepared faculty. These Hallmarks can serve as criteria to assist educators in developing career targets and benchmarks, and guide nursing programs in evaluating hiring goals, establishing annual review metrics, and supporting faculty development.

The Hallmarks and Indicators (NLN, 2020) depict well-prepared faculty as knowledgeable academic leaders committed to teaching excellence, inclusion, continuous improvement, and student engagement. As role models, well-prepared faculty support the unique mission of the nursing program and provide mentorship to students and colleagues. Well-prepared faculty engage in scholarship by practicing evidence-based teaching and clinical practice and contribute to the science of nursing through inquiry, research, presentations, and publications. Outside of the classroom, they are recognized as leaders who are actively involved in community programs, professional organizations, and interprofessional teams. Well-prepared faculty share many characteristics with another group of faculty who represent excellence and distinction — master teachers.

McMillian-Bohler et al. (2020) described master teachers as educators who possess clinical and pedagogical knowledge and exhibit an infectious passion for course content and students' learning. Master teachers are excellent communicators able to translate the most complicated concepts into accessible information for students. Master teachers are also effective in keeping students engaged in the learning process. Excellence is a continuous process (Valiga, 2010), and master teachers are vigilant in updating and improving their teaching and willingly share their expertise and missteps through scholarship and mentorship.

Constructing a cadre of well-prepared faculty who lead academic programs toward distinction and excellence requires continuous effort from individual educators and support from academic programs. According to the Hallmarks (NLN, 2020), nursing programs can support the development of well-prepared faculty by ensuring faculty are oriented and prepared for the educator role. Academic programs can assist faculty to become and remain well-prepared by providing mentors and establishing recommendations for competencies that should be achieved and maintained. The Hallmarks also posit that programs should recognize and reward faculty who contribute to the mission and vision of the school through their teaching, scholarship, and service. A significant revision to the Hallmarks as they relate to faculty is the acknowledgment that achieving excellence, distinction, and being well-prepared in nursing education requires a diverse faculty team.

THE VALUE OF FACULTY DIVERSITY

Within the NLN *Core Values* (n.d.), diversity is described in the broadest sense including the full spectrum of race, gender, ability, gender identity, culture, religion, sexual orientation, and professional experience. Faculty diversity drives innovation and contributes to the creation of a rich learning environment that enhances students' social development and the overall work environment by introducing varied and rich perspectives into curriculum and policy development, program management, and program evaluation (NLN, n.d.). Learning to value and work with persons from different backgrounds and ideologies is an important step in reducing bias and inequities and improving the quality of health care (MacDaniel, 2020).

First, racial and ethnic diversity is critical in recruiting and retaining faculty, creating an inclusive learning environment, and preparing students for clinical practice. According to the 2014 U.S. Census results (U.S. Census Bureau, 2015), underrepresented minority groups represent 38 percent of the population in the United States, yet only 20 percent of registered nurses identify as an underrepresented minority (National Council of State Boards of Nursing [NCSBN], 2018) and only 15.9 percent of nurse faculty identify as an underrepresented minority (American Association of Colleges of Nursing [AACN], 2017). Most patients are cared for by someone who does not share their culture, race, or background; this factor is associated with decreased quality of care (Degazon & Mancha, 2012). Increasing workforce diversity improves the quality of care for minority patients; however, a diverse workforce of nurses can be achieved only by increasing the diversity of nursing students. Faculty diversity improves the recruitment and retention of minority faculty (Kolade, 2016) and students from underrepresented groups (Green, 2020). Students perceive greater support and a sense of belonging, and they are more engaged when working with faculty members who look like them or share similar cultural and life experiences. Students who do not identify as belonging to an underrepresented group can also benefit from the opportunity to learn from a diverse faculty alongside peers from diverse backgrounds as they learn to work with patients from different racial and ethnic identities.

Next, other types of diversity among faculty, including gender, gender identity culture, ability, age, socioeconomic background, and other personal experiences, are also important. Diversity allows us to see our individual, unique contributions and appreciate the influence and experiences of others (NLN, 2017). Retaining a diverse faculty fosters an environment of inclusion and prepares nursing students to provide optimal care to the diverse population of patients they will encounter in their future practice. Experience working with people representing diverse experiences will also help students to master the skills required to effectively collaborate with diverse healthcare teams (Chicca & Shellenbarger, 2020).

Finally, beyond the diversity of identity and personal experience is professional diversity. Nurse educators represent a broad range of experience in education, specialty, service, scholarship, and credentials. Some faculty are expert teachers, while other faculty may be expert researchers/scientists, grant writers, clinicians, or community liaisons. Each faculty will bring unique perspectives and contribute in different ways to planning and innovation. As a complement to the Hallmarks, the *NLN Core Competencies for Nurse Educators©* (Halstead, 2018) outlines eight core competencies for nursing faculty that describe in detail the skills needed for faculty to become well-prepared.

CORE COMPETENCIES OF NURSE EDUCATORS

In 2007 (Halstead), the NLN disseminated a list of eight core competencies for nurse educators, competencies that were formulated based on an extensive review of the literature related to the roles and responsibilities of academic educators. Those competencies, updated in 2018 (Halstead), continue to guide nurse educator practice and consist of the following: Facilitate Learning, Facilitate Learner Development and Socialization, Use Effective Assessment and Evaluation Strategies, Participate in Curriculum Design and Evaluation of Program Outcomes, Function as a Change Agent and Leader, Pursue Continuous Quality Improvement in the Nurse Educator Role, Engage in Scholarship, and Function within the Educational Environment.

Competency 1: Facilitate Learning

Students must do the work of learning, but nurse educators are key to their learning process (Halstead, 2018). Nursing is a practice profession and most nursing faculty have honed expert knowledge through practice, collaboration, and scholarship in a particular clinical specialty or other areas (e.g., maternity, pediatrics, adult health, geriatrics, critical care, research, leadership, or informatics). What distinguishes master teachers (and well-prepared faculty), however, is the ability of the faculty to help students to acquire, understand, and apply content knowledge to clinical practice (McMillian-Bohler et al., 2020). An understanding of adult learning theory guides the development of lesson plans to maximize learning. There is no question that nursing students learn assessment and procedural skills in nursing school; however, critical thinking, effective communication, and prioritization are essential for high-quality nursing practice (van Wyngaarden et al., 2019). Faculty who wish to achieve excellence must possess knowledge of teaching strategies, educational technology, learning theory, and collaboration to assist students in grasping and applying these complex concepts.

To reach a variety of learners, well-prepared educators are versed in different teaching and learning strategies and modalities (e.g., effective lecturing, case studies, simulation, role-play, etc.). Not only do they know how to use technology to enhance their teaching, but they also know when to do so. It is also important to note that being well-prepared in one setting does not necessarily translate to other areas of teaching. As discovered during the rapid move to online teaching during the COVID-19 pandemic, online education and face-to-face education require a slightly different set of skills to facilitate students' learning. As noted in a review article by Collier (2018), clinical education may require yet another skill set. An in-depth discussion of teaching that facilitates excellence is available in Chapter 7.

In addition to being knowledgeable, well-prepared faculty are effective communicators, who can convey complex information to students in an accessible and appropriate manner. A communication style that conveys competence, confidence, empathy, and integrity helps to establish trust between students and faculty. Faculty must create an environment where students feel "safe" to question, explore, and learn; and they must function as role models of cultural intelligence and inclusive teaching so that all students have an opportunity to learn.

Competency 2: Facilitate Learner Development and Socialization

The Hallmarks address how faculty assist with the process of metacognition – how students think about their thinking and how the nurse educator helps students to develop as professional nurses. Well-prepared faculty share the skills necessary to develop clinical reasoning and successfully learn content. Faculty also assist students to understand the values of the profession that distinguish nursing from other professions.

More than simply giving information, the well-prepared faculty guide students in developing an approach for learning nursing concepts. By modeling how the faculty themselves work through patient scenarios, analyze evidence to determine best practice, or participate during interprofessional team meetings and rounds, students learn clinical reasoning. Faculty can explain the scaffolding process of learning with Bloom's taxonomy so that students can then use the taxonomy prompts independently to assess their level of understanding of concepts (McGuire, 2015). Using affective assignments such as reflections, faculty can help students explore the personal values that drive their decision-making and analyze how their values may change over time.

As mentors, nursing faculty also role model professionalism in nursing. Nurses have been the most trusted profession each year since 2011 (Reinhart, 2020) and faculty are in a position to be exemplars for exhibiting compassion, communicating therapeutically, utilizing evidence, maintaining a positive attitude, and practicing with integrity. Students are likely to copy what they observe. Students may also learn how to engage in self-reflection, accept feedback, or recognize and address their own biases from observing faculty. Well-prepared faculty support students as they consider new perspectives, discuss controversial topics such as bias and inequities, explore challenging ideas, and engage in difficult conversations (Clark, 2019), all of which are essential if students are to develop as compassionate, competent, confident professionals.

Competency 3: Use Effective Assessment and Evaluation Strategies

Effective assessment and evaluation provide not only a measurement of learning and preparation for practice; they also serve as a source of motivation for students and educators. Standardized testing and multiple-choice questions have long been utilized for assessment purposes in nursing education, but well-prepared, knowledgeable educators employ a variety of methods to assess student learning and identify their strengths and areas in need of improvement as they prepare for end-of-program national exams and future practice. Such methods are discussed in Chapter 7 and include competency-based simulation, written assignments, presentations, contributions to classroom or online discussions, group projects, or other scholarly work. Well-prepared faculty must know which methods to select to measure attainment of various learning objectives, design the evaluation methods thoughtfully, establish clear criteria to evaluate performance, and provide feedback to students that is both constructive and motivational. Such skills take time and deliberative action, and they develop over time, particularly as educators remain current regarding evidence to support the effective use of various approaches to assessing and evaluating learning.

Competency 4: Participate in Curriculum Design and Evaluation of Program Outcomes

Informed by essential accreditation standards and practice guidelines, as well as basic principles and tenets of curriculum design, faculty design curricula that serve as road maps for how student learning experiences will be selected and organized. Since practice, technology, the role of the nurse, and student needs change over time, faculty must remain abreast of best-evidence research related to curriculum design, essential content to be included, and effective methods to implement the curriculum if excellence is to be achieved. Thus, curriculum development and implementation, along with program evaluation, should be an ongoing component of professional faculty development.

Competency 5: Function as a Change Agent and Leader

Well-prepared faculty are in a prime position to impact nursing education, nursing practice, and the community. As academic leaders, nursing faculty can facilitate changes in curriculum, program culture, and program policy toward a preferred future (Halstead, 2018). To be an effective agent for change, well-prepared faculty must remain attentive to needs for change, thoughtful about the impact of innovation, and careful to ensure that changes align with the needs of their students, the vision of their program, and the mission of their institution. As change agents, faculty may assume the role of the innovator who creates a new approach, the early adopter who is willing to pilot new ideas and integrate them into existing educational structures, or the champion who encourages and assists others to implement changes. As role models for students and peers, the well-prepared nurse educator should also be willing and prepared to discuss, lead, and support change related to social issues such as health inequities and antidiscrimination.

The well-prepared faculty also challenges students to consider healthcare practices in the context of social and physical challenges.

The *Code of Ethics for Nurses* (American Nurses Association [ANA], 2015) calls for nurses to be patient advocates. As members of professional organizations, practicing nurses, and scholars, the well-prepared faculty can impact and lead changes in best practice and policies that impact health care. Well-prepared faculty can promote best practice on the clinical unit or as policies within a professional organization. Well-prepared faculty can also bring attention to and offer solutions for issues in the community through research and advocacy.

Competency 6: Pursue Continuous Quality Improvement in the Nurse Educator Role

The Hallmarks indicate that well-prepared faculty are consistently engaged in continuous learning and improvement. The needs of students and patients and advances in health care and technology are constantly evolving. In response to the dynamic nature of teaching and practice, the well-prepared faculty engages in lifelong learning related to content and teaching. For example, simulation, including high fidelity mannequin and standardized patients, has been rapidly integrated into learning and evaluation, and it is now a valid replacement for a percentage of hospital clinical experiences. Students expect simulation to be a part of their training, and faculty have learned to integrate new teaching frameworks, vocabularies, and tools into their repertoire. Well-prepared faculty should not only expect to update their teaching regularly, but they should also be excited by the prospect of continuously improving their craft. Well-prepared faculty elicit feedback from students, peers, and administrators to make positive changes. They attend conferences on teaching and learning, read books and articles, listen to podcasts, and follow by any means available news of breakthroughs in the classroom because they enjoy and are dedicated to teaching excellence. During the Coronavirus pandemic, well-prepared faculty worked to improve accessibility and to enrich their courses each semester, explored virtual learning options, and addressed student needs despite unprecedented challenges to teaching and learning environments. Well-prepared faculty constantly ask what can be done better.

Competency 7: Engage in Scholarship

The purpose of scholarship is to improve practice and provide documentation of excellence and an essential responsibility of nurse faculty (Kalensky & Hande, 2017). In 1990, Boyer expanded the definition of scholarship to include not only the creation of new knowledge but innovative teaching, interprofessional work, and sharing outside the home institution. As a practice profession, scholarship in nursing must be broadly defined to be accessible to educators in a variety of settings. In 2018, the AACN identified three pillars of scholarship in nursing education: practice, teaching, and discovery. According to AACN, scholarship or practice is evident in the consistent application of evidence in practice. Scholarship of practice is also the spirit of inquiry that compels the nurse to investigate ways to improve the quality of care. The scholarship of teaching can include the application of evidence to the work of teaching, but it can also include exploring ways to be innovative and sharing findings and new ideas with other faculty. The scholarship of discovery includes not only traditional empirical research, but historical and philosophical inquiry, methodological studies, and theory development (AACN, 1999). Furthermore, scholarship of discovery can take the form of publications, mentorship, or presentations. Ultimately, the activities that define acceptable and expected scholarship vary among institutions and the well-prepared faculty will ensure that their skill set and interest are aligned with the requirements set forth by their home institution.

Competency 8: Function within the Educational Environment

The learning environment is influenced by many factors, including the mission, vision, and core values of the college/school or university; state and national laws and regulations; and the cultural climate of the learning institution. For example, an institution may be particularly focused on obtaining national funding, building community programming, or supporting students from diverse backgrounds. Well-prepared faculty must be aware of influences on the learning environment and be able to integrate them successfully into their teaching, mentoring, and scholarship. Well-prepared faculty should, therefore, select their parent institution thoughtfully to ensure that their professional interests and values are aligned with those of their employer.

HALLMARKS OF EXCELLENCE AS THEY RELATE TO FACULTY

The NLN Hallmarks (NLN, 2020), along with the Indicators for each, can serve as guidelines to assist faculty in establishing career goals and benchmarks, and guide nursing programs in evaluating hiring goals, establishing annual review metrics, and supporting faculty development that is associated with achieving distinction in nursing.

Well-prepared faculty are critical to the achievement of excellence and distinction in nursing education; therefore, nursing programs must support the ongoing development of faculty regarding their competencies as educators. The five Hallmarks related to diverse, well-prepared faculty and the 16 Indicators related to them help schools clarify the goals toward which they need to work to create and sustain a faculty complement that maximizes its diversity and embraces a commitment to excellence as educators. These Hallmarks can be used to determine hiring criteria; formulate approaches to, and criteria for, annual faculty evaluations; influence promotion and tenure criteria; and establish strategic goals for the school.

Faculty Are Diverse Leaders and Experts

Schools/colleges of nursing should have a public statement of commitment to hiring faculty who are diverse regarding their backgrounds, passions, and areas of expertise, as well as a specific plan for achieving such diversity in hiring. By having such a diverse group of educators, students can interact and learn with faculty who look and think differently, and who exhibit various strengths and passions. Such a group also contributes to more thoughtful discussions where a wide range of possibilities are considered before decisions are made, and it provides opportunities for the school to excel in many ways. The outcome of such diversity, therefore, benefits students, faculty, and the entire school, and it facilitates the achievement of excellence and distinction.

Faculty Contributions Are Valued, Rewarded, and Recognized

Although faculty in any type of institution – research-intensive, teaching-intensive, service/ community-oriented – often find it challenging to balance the demands of teaching, service, practice, and scholarship, expectations in all these areas typically are placed on all faculty. The extent of contributions in each area is likely to vary based on the institution's mission, the faculty member's area of expertise and passion, the strategic goals of the school/college of nursing, professional goals of individuals, or any number of other factors. This Hallmark asserts that no matter what an individual's major contributions are to the overall academic effort, they should be valued, recognized, and rewarded. Schools need excellent and passionate teachers, accomplished scholars, leaders in professional organizations, community builders, and individuals who do the day-to-day work of the school if they are to achieve distinction; thus, no one category of expertise or passion should be any more important, "spotlighted" more, or rewarded more than the other categories. Schools might consider the faculty awards they give, the expectations that exist for faculty to receive merit raises, the opportunities provided to all faculty to be involved at the university/college level or to participate in special initiatives, and other factors so that no one group feels disenfranchised or taken for granted and not valued. It is by recognizing, rewarding, and visibly valuing the various contributions made by faculty that a healthy workplace will evolve, and excellence can be achieved.

Faculty Promote Excellence, Create Inclusive Environments, and Provide Leadership

The burden of creating a healthful work environment or enhancing the school's reputation does not rest solely with the academic administrator. Indeed, those responsibilities are shared among administrators, students, and faculty, and it is the faculty who are in an excellent position to lead the way. Research has documented the extensiveness of incivility in schools of nursing (Clark, 2019), incivility that exists among students, between students and faculty, among faculty, and between faculty and administrators. Incivility can negatively impact the teaching and learning environment (Clark & Springer, 2010), increase student's stress and lead to further acts of incivility with peers and faculty, and decrease overall program satisfaction (Marchiondo et al., 2010). Faculty can collaborate with one another, as well as with students and administrators, to establish codes of conduct for the school with particular programs (e.g., pre-licensure, master's), and/or for individual courses where all those involved are expected to be respectful, inclusive, honest, transparent, willing to address uncivil behaviors when they occur, and enforce a zero-tolerance policy for racism, bullying, and discrimination in classrooms, laboratories, clinical sites, and all avenues of research and scholarship. Examples include the Rutgers School of Nursing standards of conduct (https://nursing .rutgers.edu/students/conduct/) and Lakeview College of Nursing's code of conduct (https://www.lakeviewcol.edu/catalog-2018-2019/section-v-policies-and-standards-behavior/code-conduct). They also can collaborate to discuss the meaning of excellence in academe and their own school, programs, and courses, thereby creating a deeper understanding of what excellence means in that context and how everyone contributes to achieving it. And faculty can function as leaders (Grossman & Valiga, 2021) who engage others in facilitating change in their areas of expertise or passion that leads to excellence and distinction. There is no question that this Hallmark recognizes the critical role faculty play in achieving excellence in nursing education.

Faculty Model Commitment to Lifelong Learning, Professional Involvement, and Scholarly Activities

Excellence is a continuous process (Valiga, 2017). To achieve excellence, faculty must revise and update curricula to ensure that they remain relevant to today's environment and prepare students for the ever-changing, uncertain, technology-infused areas in which they will practice. Students also evolve, and to maintain excellence, nurse educators must be dedicated to updating the strategies they use to meet the learning needs of an increasingly diverse student body. Research continues to inform us of the most effective practice standards and approaches to facilitate learning, so faculty must stay current to engage in evidence-based teaching and clinical practice, and they must participate in building the science that underlies both arenas of practice. Finally, the challenges facing our profession continue to change, so active involvement in professional organizations that address those challenges and help shape the future of our profession is essential for faculty to be part of such efforts. There is no question, then, that one of the factors essential to achieving excellence in nursing education is a faculty complement that engages in lifelong learning – about clinical phenomena and pedagogical approaches – that is involved professionally, and that engages in scholarly work. Not only do such efforts contribute to effective programs and advance the profession of nursing, but they also serve as a way for faculty to serve as role models for students and one another.

Faculty Have Structured Preparation for the Faculty Role

Most faculty teaching in today's schools/colleges of nursing are prepared as clinicians, not educators. They are comfortable in the practice setting and confident in their clinical knowledge and skills and often are at Benner's (2000, p. 31) level of expert in that role. However, they have had little to no preparation for the role in which they are now engaged – that of an educator.

The nurse educator competencies discussed earlier clarify how complex and multifaceted the role of an academic educator is, yet few faculty are prepared to fulfill those expectations. In essence, they are novices in this role and must first make the transition from expert (clinician) to novice (educator) before they can make the transition from novice to expert educator or master teacher.

If schools are to achieve excellence in nursing education, then faculty must be prepared for the complex role they assume on appointment. That preparation could occur through formal academic programs, continuing education programs/workshops, participation in academies or teaching fellowships, or deliberate mentoring from a master teacher; and it is enhanced by purposeful self-study, reading education-focused books and journals, preparation for the Certified Nurse Educator (CNE®) examination (http://www.nln.org/Certification-for-Nurse-Educators/cne/eligibility), and careful self-reflection of one's strengths and areas in need of improvement as an educator. With such effort on the part of individuals – and supported by the school in which they are employed – faculty can become increasingly competent as educators and some may even become master teachers — most certainly a mark of distinction.

CONCLUSION

Nurses comprise the largest contingency of the healthcare system (Institute of Medicine [IOM], 2011), and for 18 years the public has identified nursing as the most trusted among a wide range of professions (Reinhart, 2020). Nurses have an immense impact on individual lives and health care in communities, and future generations of nurses must be prepared to meet the demands and responsibilities of this trusted role. Such a goal will be achieved through the efforts of well-prepared nurse educators who create curricula, design and implement strategies to facilitate and evaluate learning, evaluate programs for their effectiveness, engage in scholarly work, participate actively in professional organizations, and provide leadership in their schools, universities, communities, and profession. As highlighted in the Hallmarks discussed here, a diverse, well-prepared faculty is fundamental to the achievement of distinction and excellence in nursing education; therefore, faculty must be dedicated to developing, nurturing, and enhancing their teaching skills and the academic institutions in which they work must provide the support and recognition needed by faculty to perform a vitally important job.

The NLN Hallmarks (2020) articulate expectations related to a diverse, well-prepared faculty that are essential to achieve distinction. Additionally, documents such as the NLN *Core Competencies* define the skills needed by all faculty to prepare nursing students to face practice in a diverse world with competence, confidence, and compassion. It is incumbent on faculty to be dedicated to achieving excellence and distinction, and universities and colleagues must be dedicated to supporting excellence through their hiring, support for development, and recognition of faculty. Patients trust nurses, and faculty must be well-prepared to help students deliver the high quality of care expected of them.

References

American Association of Colleges of Nursing. (1999). *Defining scholarship for the discipline of nursing*. https://www.aacnnursing.org/News-Information/Position-Statements-White-Papers/Defining-Scholarship

American Association of Colleges of Nursing. (2017). *Nursing faculty: A spotlight on diversity*. https://www.aacnnursing.org/portals/42/policy/pdf/diversity-spotlight.pdf

American Association of Colleges of Nursing. (2018). *Defining scholarship* for academic nursing: Task force consensus position statement. http://www.aacnnursing.org/News-Information/Position-Statements-White-Papers/Defining-Scholarship-Nursing

American Nurses Association. (2015). *Code of ethics for nurses with interpretive statements.* Nursesbooks.org. https://www.nursingworld.org/practice-policy/nursing-excellence/ethics/code-of-ethics-for-nurses/coe-view-only/

Benner, P. (2000). *From novice to expert.* Pearson.

Billings, D. M., & Halstead, J. A. (2019). *Teaching in nursing: A guide for faculty* (6th ed.). Elsevier.

Booth, T. L., Emerson, C. J., Hackney, M. G., & Souter, S. (2016). Preparation of academic nurse educators. *Nurse Education in Practice, 19,* 54–57. https://doi.org/10.1016/j.nepr.2016.04.006

Chicca, J., & Shellenbarger, T. (2020). Fostering inclusive clinical learning environments using a psychological safety lens. *Teaching and Learning in Nursing, 15*(4), 226–232. https://doi-org.proxy.lib.duke.edu/10.1016/j.teln.2020.03.002

Christensen, L. S., & Simmons, L. E. (2019). *The scope of practice for academic nurse educators and academic clinical nurse educators* (3rd ed.). National League for Nursing.

Clark, C. M. (2019). Fostering a culture of civility and respect in nursing. *Journal of Nursing Regulation, 10*(1), 44–52. https://doi.org/10.1016/S2155-8256(19)30082-1

Clark, C. M., & Springer, P. J. (2010). Academic nurse leaders' role in fostering a culture of civility in nursing education. *The Journal of Nursing Education, 49*(6), 319–325. https://doi.org/10.3928/01484834-20100224-01

Collier, A. D. (2018). Characteristics of an effective nursing clinical instructor: The state of the science. *Journal of Clinical Nursing, 27*(1-2), 363–374. https://doi.org/10.1111/jocn.13931

Degazon, C. E., & Mancha, C. (2012). Changing the face of nursing: Reducing ethnic and racial disparities in health. *Family and Community Health, 35*(1), 5–14. https://doi.org/10.1097/FCH.0b013e3182385cf6

Green, C. (2020). Equity and diversity in nursing education. *Teaching and Learning in Nursing, 15*(4), 280–283. https://doi.org/10.1016/j.teln.2020.07.004

Grossman, S., & Valiga, T. (2021). *The new leadership challenge: Creating a preferred future* (6th ed.). F.A. Davis.

Halstead, J. (2007). *Nurse educator competencies: Creating an evidence-based practice for nurse educators.* National League for Nursing.

Halstead, J. A. (Ed.). (2018). *NLN core competencies for nurse educators: A decade of influence.* National League for Nursing.

Institute of Medicine. (2011). *The future of nursing: Leading change, advancing health.* National Academies Press. https://www.nap.edu/catalog/12956/the-future-of-nursing-leading-change-advancing-health

Kalensky, M., & Hande, K. (2017). Transition from expert clinician to novice faculty: A blueprint for success. *Journal for Nurse Practitioners, 13*(9), e433–e439. https://doi-org.proxy.lib.duke.edu/10.1016/j.nurpra.2017.06.005

Kolade, F. M. (2016). The lived experience of minority nursing faculty: A phenomenological study. *Journal of Professional Nursing, 32*(2), 107–114. https://doi-org.proxy.lib.duke.edu/10.1016/j.profnurs.2015.09.002

MacDaniel, T. E. (2020). Enhancing learning in diverse classrooms to improve nursing practice. *Teaching and Learning in Nursing, 15*(4), 245–247. https://doi.org/10.1016/j.teln.2020.05.004

Marchiondo, K., Marchiondo, L. A., & Lasiter, S. (2010). Faculty incivility: Effects on program satisfaction of BSN students. *Journal of Nursing Education, 49*(11), 608–614. https://doi.org/10.3928/01484834-20100524-05

McGuire, S. (2015). *Teach students how to learn.* Stylus Publishing.

McMillian-Bohler, J., Copel, L., & Todd-Magel, C. (2020). A description of the characteristics and behaviors of master teachers in nursing. *International Journal of Nursing Education Scholarship, 18*(1), 1–10. https://doi.org/10.1515/ijnes-2018-0044

National Council of State Boards of Nursing. (2018). *2017 RN practice analysis: Linking the NCLEX-RN examination to practice U.S. and Canada.* https://www.ncsbn.org/17_RN_US_Canada_Practice_Analysis.pdf

National League for Nursing. (2017). *NLN program outcomes and competencies for graduate academic nurse educator preparation.* http://www.nln.org/docs/default-source/professional-development-programs/program-outcomes-and-competencies2.pdf?sfvrsn=2

National League for Nursing. (2020). *Hallmarks of excellence in nursing education.* http://www.nln.org/docs/default-source/default-document-library/hallmarks_of_excellence_2019.pdf?sfvrsn=0

National League for Nursing. (n.d.). *Core values.* http://www.nln.org/about/core-values

Reinhart, R. J. (2020). *Nurses continue to rate high in honest, ethics,* https://news.gallup.com/poll/274673/nurses-continue-rate-highest-honesty-ethics.aspx

United States Census Bureau. (2015). *New Census Bureau report analyzes U.S. population projections.* https://www.census.gov/newsroom/press-releases/2015/cb15-tps16.html#:~:text=The%20minority%20population%20is%20projected,will%20actually%20occur%20in%202029

Valiga T. M. (2010). Excellence — Does the word mean anything anymore? *Journal of Nursing Education, 49*(8), 427–428. https://doi.org/10.3928/01484834-20100721-01

Valiga, T. M. (2017). Do schools of nursing truly value excellence in teaching? Actions speak louder than words. *Journal of Nursing Education, 56,* 519–520. https://doi.org/10.3928/01484834-20170817-01

van Wyngaarden, A., Leech, R., & Coetzee, I. (2019). Challenges nurse educators experience with development of student nurses' clinical reasoning skills. *Nurse Education in Practice, 40.* https://doi-org.proxy.lib.duke.edu/10.1016/j.nepr.2019.102623

World Health Organization. (2016). *Nurse educator competencies.* https://www.who.int/hrh/nursing_midwifery/nurse_educator050416.pdf

5

Achieving Distinction Through a Culture of Continuous Quality Improvement

Judith A. Halstead, PhD, RN, CNE, FAAN, ANEF

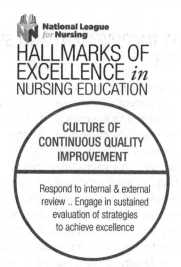

National League for Nursing

HALLMARKS OF EXCELLENCE *in* NURSING EDUCATION

CULTURE OF CONTINUOUS QUALITY IMPROVEMENT

Respond to internal & external review .. Engage in sustained evaluation of strategies to achieve excellence

INTRODUCTION

Nursing faculty and program administrators are responsible and accountable to stakeholders for ensuring the educational quality that exists within the student learning environments in our schools/colleges of nursing. Students, faculty, program and institution administrators, healthcare employers, regulatory bodies, the nursing profession, and ultimately our patients are representative of the diverse stakeholders whose interests are best served by high-quality nursing programs. These stakeholders are vested in having confidence that nursing programs will consistently produce competent nurses prepared to meet the challenges of delivering care in complex and uncertain healthcare systems. Accepting the responsibility to ensure a high level of educational quality requires faculty and administrators to be intentional and systematic in their efforts to create an educational environment infused with an ongoing focus of being the "best that one can be." Creating an organizational culture of continuous quality improvement (CQI) helps administrators and faculty achieve the outcomes necessary for the program to demonstrate excellence and achieve distinction.

The purpose of this chapter is to describe how nursing faculty and administrators can create an environment in which a culture of CQI flourishes and facilitates the ongoing program review and revision designed to meet the following Hallmarks of Excellence in Nursing Education© disseminated by the National League for Nursing (NLN): *Program design, implementation, and evaluation are continuously reviewed and revised to achieve and maintain excellence.* (All Hallmarks and the Indicators for each are included as Appendix B.) The importance of designing an evidence-based program evaluation process that is inclusive of faculty, staff, students, and other stakeholder feedback is emphasized. The use of strategic planning processes that facilitate meeting the program's mission with quality and excellence also is addressed, as is the value of seeking national nursing accreditation.

CONTINUOUS QUALITY IMPROVEMENT AND SYSTEMATIC PROGRAM EVALUATION

The processes of continuous quality improvement (CQI) and systematic program evaluation (SPE) have a number of overarching purposes in common. While engaging in CQI represents the faculty's commitment to the pursuit of excellence, engaging in SPE provides faculty with a framework and structure by which to organize and apply meaning to their CQI endeavors. However, implementing the CQI and SPE processes effectively requires institutions and programs to establish the organizational culture expectations associated with successful implementation efforts.

Understanding the purposes and requirements of CQI and SPE also provides the foundation for faculty to achieve the quality Indicators associated with the following Hallmark: *The program engages in a variety of activities that promote quality and excellence, including accreditation by national nursing accreditation bodies.* CQI and SPE are the processes needed for faculty to successfully develop a mechanism by which to participate in the continuous review of program design, implementation, and evaluation, and to ensure that program decision-making is based on findings from ongoing review efforts. Respectful use of data and transparent decision-making that engages all stakeholders are ways that faculty can be engaged with administrators in quality improvement efforts.

What are the purposes for nursing faculty and administrators to pursue CQI and SPE? First, both processes provide the program with the opportunity to demonstrate to their internal and external stakeholders that they are committed to program quality and excellence. The intentionality of their efforts become apparent to others who are also vested in the program's outcomes.

Second, both CQI and SPE provide the faculty with opportunities to highlight their program's effectiveness and areas of strength or uniqueness, as well as identify areas that need improvement. Using these processes together allow the faculty to answer questions such as the following: "How can we do what we do, even better?" and "What areas of our program would benefit from additional attention and resources to achieve the desired outcomes?" CQI and SPE are data-driven processes that require faculty to gather and analyze data before determining an intervention plan.

A third common purpose associated with both CQI and SPE is the use of these processes to provide data and a rationale to use when requesting additional resources. Obtaining grant funds, increasing budget allocations for project implementation, and securing donors to support program initiatives can be direct outcomes of the faculty systematically analyzing data, determining program needs, and creating an evidence-based financial request that will resonate with potential funders. Programs that have achieved a reputation for distinction among their peers will typically have a strong history of resource acquisition from internal and external stakeholders who believe in the program's mission and want to play a role in supporting the continuing success of the program.

The successful implementation of the CQI and SPE processes also has associated organizational expectations necessary to create an environment in which quality improvement efforts can flourish and be sustained. It is not possible for faculty to successfully pursue excellence in all elements of the program if an ongoing commitment to quality is not evident at both the institutional and programmatic levels. A recent study conducted by the National Council of State Boards of Nursing (NCSBN) reported two emerging themes that suggested program vulnerability to decreased performance outcomes was related to a lack of administrative processes being in place and the inability to use data in program decision-making (Spector et al., 2020). A lack of quality improvement processes related to program evaluation was one of the examples of administrative processes given. In addition, the authors stated that even when data was collected by the program, there was evidence that faculty were not prepared to interpret the data. Given such evidence, it is critical that programs demonstrate a visible commitment to quality. There are many ways such a commitment can be made visible. Allocating fiscal and human resources are obvious examples of commitment; additional examples include highlighting outcomes associated with successful CQI efforts, providing faculty with opportunities to develop competencies related to their role in program evaluation, and fostering a constructive approach to addressing data findings associated with evaluation.

Another expectation is that there is a good-faith effort exhibited by faculty and administration related to the program's self-assessment of program strengths and areas for improvement, with a genuine interest in collecting data and sharing the findings with the appropriate stakeholders. For some, the evaluation process can be perceived to be a threatening force, associated with a fear of potential change, but transparency about what is done well and what needs improvement is essential if a healthful, open, and supportive environment is to be created and sustained.

Individuals need to be able to trust that there will be no fault-finding or criticism associated with the process of data collection and analysis. To encourage buy-in and participation in quality improvement efforts, it is essential that there be a respectful use of all evaluation data as the findings are disseminated. A commitment to transparency in decision-making as the data are analyzed and used to make program changes is another important requirement. The feedback mechanisms that will be used need to be clearly defined and disseminated to all involved parties.

And, finally, it is essential to emphasize that successful quality improvement efforts require the engagement of all. CQI is not a "top-down" initiative or one that is delegated to a particular individual alone; rather, it is one that enthusiastically seeks to invite the participation of all stakeholders as program evaluation efforts are undertaken.

CREATING A CULTURE OF CONTINUOUS QUALITY IMPROVEMENT IN NURSING EDUCATION

Implementing the CQI process within nursing education requires faculty and administrators to commit to ongoing self-assessment through which they collect and analyze data, and then use those data to identify evidence-based strategies for program improvement (Ellis & Halstead, 2012). To adequately measure program effectiveness, the process used to collect, analyze, and disseminate data needs to consistently and systematically address all elements of the program deemed essential to meeting the expected program outcomes (see Box 5-1).

Professional standards, guidelines, and accreditation standards can be used to provide a systematic framework for program evaluation. The NLN Hallmarks also provide a comprehensive framework that can be used to inform faculty dialogue about what actions can lead to excellence for their program. (The Self-Assessment Checklist included as Appendix C can help guide such dialogue.) However, even with all these guiding tools available to faculty, use of them alone will not create success. To successfully engage in CQI and move a program toward recognized distinction, it is important for faculty and administrators to first create an organizational environment within which the culture of CQI can be established, celebrated, and allowed to flourish.

As the name implies, CQI is an ongoing process with established feedback mechanisms that allow faculty and administrators to systematically examine the program's goals and expected outcomes for relevance, appropriateness, and effectiveness. Are the goals relevant to the current and projected future practice environment? Are the stated goals appropriate to the degree being pursued (PN/VN, ADN, BSN, MSN, DNP, and/or PhD)? Are the goals being met? Is the program achieving the desired outcomes? What program outcome trends are emerging from the data analyses, and are those trends headed in the desired direction? For example, are licensing and certification pass rates, completion rates, and employment rates meeting established benchmarks? Should the goals and expected outcomes be adjusted to enhance program quality and

---

BOX 5-1

Program Elements

Program Outcomes (licensure/certification pass rates, completion rates, graduation rates, employment rates, etc.)

- Mission, Goals, Governance
- Institutional and Program Resources
- Faculty and Staff
- Students
- Curriculum and Evaluation Processes

Source: Boland, 2015; Ellis, 2020

BOX 5-2

Creating a Culture of Continuous Quality Improvement

- Establish clear goals, expected outcomes
- Address the needs of constituents
- Define benchmarks of success
- Collect, analyze, and use data for decision-making
- Ensure a collaborative process
- Engage in collective decision-making

---

better meet the needs of identified stakeholders? Where is the program most successful in achieving its goals and outcomes, and what areas require some focused attention for improvement? The cultural foundations of CQI that must be integrated into the environment to foster program excellence can be found in Box 5-2 and are further described in the following paragraphs.

Establishing Goals and Expected Outcomes

To determine if program goals and expected outcomes are being met, it is essential that faculty and administrators first establish clear goals and expected program outcomes against which to measure progress. Expected program outcomes can be defined as "anticipated outcomes established by faculty and staff accompanied by associated benchmark measures used by the program to determine if the outcome has been met" (NLN Commission for Nursing Education Accreditation [CNEA], 2016, p. 35). In this context, program goals and outcomes are all-encompassing of the various program elements (see Box 5-1). For example, the program faculty will want to set goals and expected outcomes associated with faculty resources and accomplishments; the curriculum and teaching/learning strategies; student learning and achievement; student support services and instructional resources; and any other Indicator of program quality that faculty, administrators, and staff deem appropriate for meeting the institution and program mission, as well as the overall success of the program (NLN CNEA, 2016).

Program goals and outcomes should be used to drive program decision-making, resource allocation, implementation strategies, and program evaluation efforts. Therefore, setting clear, measurable program goals and expected outcomes is an indispensable first step in the CQI process. Goals and outcomes should be mission aligned and include aspiration goals that will facilitate the program achieving excellence and distinction in its self-identified areas of desired accomplishments. How does the program want to be recognized by external constituencies? How will program success be measured? How will the needs of various stakeholders be addressed?

Addressing the Needs of Stakeholders

Identifying meaningful program goals and expected outcomes requires faculty and administrators to engage in a thoughtful, self-reflective process at regular intervals to systematically discuss and determine how to best uphold or refine the program's mission and address the needs of stakeholders. For example, it is critical that the program understands the demographics of its student population and their learning needs. The practice needs of healthcare partners and the employers who hire the program's graduates should also be taken into consideration. Faculty and staff role development needs must be identified along with the resources required to address them. Keeping the curriculum and teaching/learning strategies relevant and up to date requires faculty to implement ongoing processes that allow them to stay current regarding pedagogical research findings, as well as societal, healthcare, and professional nursing trends that will influence curriculum development. The process of identifying program priorities and addressing stakeholder needs should flow from these discussions, allowing faculty and administrators to set relevant goals and expected outcomes.

A culture of CQI will foster an environment in which faculty and administrators regularly and actively seek input and feedback from stakeholders to inform program decision-making. Programs that desire to achieve distinction for their accomplishments will always demonstrate a keen understanding of the needs of their stakeholders and strive to design initiatives to meet those needs.

Defining Benchmarks of Success

Another Hallmark of successful implementation of the CQI process is for the faculty to set standards, or benchmarks, by which to measure the program's effectiveness in achieving expected outcomes. Benchmarks are assigned to the program elements that are identified by faculty as being essential to determining the success of the program and defining its excellence. For example, benchmarks can be set related to student outcomes (e.g., licensure/certification pass rates, completion rates, and graduate employment), faculty accomplishments, student support, instructional resources, curricular outcomes, and so on.

To demonstrate excellence in outcomes and achieve distinction, the benchmarks set by faculty should be realistic, yet aspirational and motivational to administrators, faculty, and students. Benchmarks should be a "fit" for the institution and program's mission, providing a focused target for all to work toward. Benchmarks also help guide the allocation of resources, as faculty must carefully consider what processes need to be implemented to successfully meet the established benchmark. See Box 5-3 for a series of questions that faculty can discuss when considering program outcome benchmarks that will help them achieve excellence.

The benchmarking process also implies that when deciding how to set the benchmark for a particular program element, a comparison is made to quality standards and evidence-based best practices that exist within the profession. Faculty can choose appropriate benchmarks by reviewing the literature for evidence-based practices that yield positive outcomes, considering accreditation standards, selecting peer institutions and programs that are recognized for demonstrating excellence and have similar missions with comparable faculty and student populations, and considering the program's student demographics. Such considerations will provide a unique dataset that faculty can use to identify realistic, mission-aligned benchmarks by which to measure their program's effectiveness.

BOX 5-3

Factors to Consider When Developing Outcome Benchmarks

- Does the program have a strategic plan in place with identified outcome goals and associated timelines?
- What are the program's priorities?
- What program outcomes do faculty want to benchmark?
- What are the program's concerns and challenges?
- What are the program's areas for growth?
- Choose a concern/issue and review the data – what is the current status? What goals, if achieved, would indicate success to faculty? What benchmark, if achieved, would be a measure of success?

Collecting, Analyzing, and Using Data

The CQI process is data-driven, requiring faculty and staff to give thoughtful consideration as to what data needs to be collected to support program quality improvement efforts. Program excellence will not be achieved if decisions are based solely upon the faculty's intuition, past practices, or inherent and unrecognized biases, lacking any evidence as to what actions to take to effectively address the program element under review. Decisions must be informed by data to be credible.

Effective decision-making to improve program quality necessitates having access to reliable data that has been collected, carefully analyzed, and used to inform faculty discussion. Data can also be used to nurture and support faculty creativity and the introduction of new and innovative strategies. Nursing programs that foster excellence and achieve distinction among their nursing academic peers often have reputations for encouraging creativity and innovation in program design and implementation, as well as having robust evaluation plans in place to measure the effectiveness of any new initiatives. Proactively anticipating the data needed to demonstrate program success or support making changes is a cornerstone to responsible program innovation, implementation, and quality improvement.

Ensuring a Collaborative Process

Another important step to building a culture of CQI to influence program excellence is for administrators and faculty to nurture a sense of engagement and shared responsibility, viewing program evaluation as a collaborative process (Halstead, 2019). A collaborative environment can be accomplished when faculty and other stakeholders are invited to participate in the data collection and analysis process, as well as provide feedback used to inform decision-making. There are many ways to foster collaboration, including open dialogue about areas of program evaluation, collaborative selection of data collection methods, dissemination of findings to stakeholders, and clear communication of the final outcomes of decision-making. Maintaining a transparent and open approach to program evaluation will increase trust and participation in the process, as well as strengthen the program's relationships with stakeholders (Halstead, 2019).

Engaging in Collective Decision-Making

The final foundational element to creating a culture of CQI is to engage in collective decision-making when addressing program issues. Decision-making in a healthy CQI environment is not a "top-down" process. Rather, it is a mission-driven, goal-centered process that gathers input, as appropriate, from those who will be affected by the decision, and carefully considers the collective perspectives of all stakeholders. When the final decision is made, the rationale for the decision will be evident to all.

SYSTEMATIC PROGRAM EVALUATION

Creating and sustaining an organizational culture that is supportive of CQI is only possible if faculty and administrators consider ways in which program design, implementation, and evaluation can be continuously reviewed and revised to achieve and maintain excellence, as noted in the Hallmarks in this area. A key faculty characteristic that exemplifies program excellence is a demonstrated willingness to regularly engage in self-assessment of the program's strengths and areas requiring attention, adjusting, and revising as necessary to implement program improvements. In the quest for excellence, what mechanism is designed by faculty and put in place to ensure the continuous review of program elements?

SPE is one process that faculty can implement to provide the organizational framework that will effectively guide them in establishing a continuous review plan of all program elements. The goal of SPE is to engage in program evaluation methods designed to systematically assess, measure, and improve the program's effectiveness in achieving expected program outcomes. The specific purposes of program evaluation are identified in Box 5-4.

The purposes of SPE cannot be achieved without a systematic and regular plan for data collection, usually captured in the systematic evaluation plan (SEP), a written document that provides faculty with a "roadmap" to evaluating program outcomes and highlighting program achievements (Halstead, 2019). The faculty should consider the SEP to be a dynamic plan, one that evaluates all program elements (see Box 5-1), reflects the program's priority outcomes, and is referenced frequently as faculty engage in program decision-making. In addition to the usual components of the SEP (outcomes to

---

BOX 5-4

Purposes of Program Evaluation

Faculty engage in program evaluation to address the following questions:
- Is the program effective in meeting the mission, goals, and program outcomes?
- Has the program been implemented as faculty planned?
- What rationale exists to guide faculty decision-making to improve program quality?
- How do program elements interact to impact program effectiveness?
- Are the necessary resources being acquired and effectively used to improve quality?

Source: Ellis, 2020

be evaluated, timelines, benchmarks, data collection methods, and assigned responsibility for data collection and analysis), the SEP should also describe how the data findings will be shared with stakeholders and used by faculty to make program decisions. Sharing the findings and seeking input from those who are vested in the program's outcomes can help build trust with the process and strengthen relationships with stakeholders (Halstead, 2019), thus further deepening the faculty's commitment to quality improvement. An SEP that is comprehensive, consistently implemented, and produces data that is used to make program improvements is key to demonstrating excellence and achieving program distinction in nursing education.

ACCREDITATION: A PUBLIC MARK OF QUALITY

CQI, SPE, and accreditation are interrelated with a common goal of ensuring program quality. All three processes involve collecting data (evidence) to demonstrate that the program is effective and efficient at achieving expected program outcomes, and to identify areas for improvement. As has been discussed, systematically collecting, analyzing, and using data to inform program decision-making are Hallmark Indicators of CQI and SPE. While CQI and SPE are more internally directed evaluation processes undertaken by the program, the accreditation process represents an opportunity for the program to earn a public mark of quality that exemplifies program excellence. It is not possible for a program to successfully pursue and maintain accreditation if a culture of CQI and a process to ensure SPE is lacking.

Accreditation has been defined as "a standards-based, evidence-based, judgement-based, peer-based process" (Eaton, 2012a, p. 14). To achieve accreditation, the program conducts an evidence-based self-assessment of program effectiveness as measured by the ability to demonstrate compliance with a set of pre-established standards, documenting the findings of this self-assessment in a self-study report. Following a review of the self-study report; participation in interviews with faculty, students, and other program stakeholders; and the review of other program documents, a team of peers render a decision as to the extent the program has successfully met the standards.

Accreditation has as its primary purpose the protection of the public, which is achieved by holding programs publicly accountable to quality and a commitment to the process of quality improvement (Eaton, 2012b). Accreditation of nursing programs has long been a voluntary activity, but in recent years increasing numbers of states have legislated that it be required. The benefits of accreditation are many (see Box 5–5) for the program and its students.

Accreditation standards can be used by faculty to guide program evaluation as it enables faculty to systematically evaluate all elements of the program. The elements of program evaluation (see Box 5-1) can be found in all accreditation standards regardless of the national nursing accreditation body, along with quality Indicators that, if achieved, exemplify excellence. Faculty can, of course, use the Hallmarks or identify additional elements to be evaluated as suited to the unique and distinctive nature of their program, and should not consider program evaluation to be limited to solely meeting accreditation standards.

BOX 5-5

Benefits of Nursing Program Accreditation

- Public acknowledgement of program quality
- Eligibility for federal or state funding to support program initiatives
- Marketability of graduates to employers
- Institutional transfer of academic credits
- Ease of academic progression for students

Source: Eaton, 2012b; Halstead, 2019

Accreditation is often said to stifle faculty innovation and creativity, thus limiting a program's ability to implement changes in response to challenges. Challenges bring "opportunities for engaging in continuous quality improvement and developing new approaches to facilitate learning and prepare graduates to practice in a complex health-care environment" (Halstead, 2020, p. A-4); accreditation can be used as a partner in meeting those challenges. Achieving accreditation requires programs to maintain a contemporary curriculum and implement innovative teaching/learning strategies that foster student achievement of learning outcomes. Accreditation requires programs to gather data to support decision-making, and a successful journey to achieving accreditation requires faculty to collectively address program issues with stakeholders. Accreditation standards also require resources to be made available to support CQI efforts and innovation. When faculty plan to implement innovative curriculum and teaching/learning strategy changes, accreditation standards support that faculty development opportunities be provided to guide faculty in the changes, as well as proactively develop evaluation plans to measure the effectiveness of the changes.

Achieving accreditation in and of itself does not automatically ensure that excellence will be reached and distinction exemplified by the program. However, participating in the accreditation process and successfully demonstrating that faculty have reached that program milestone does provide a solid foundation upon which faculty can continue to engage in creative and innovative ways to foster student success, ultimately earning the mark of distinction. The NLN Hallmarks provide a model that faculty can use to continue to nurture program creativity and innovation beyond the expectations of the accreditation process, by setting Hallmark benchmarks for achieving excellence and distinction. When faculty integrate the NLN Hallmarks into their CQI efforts, along with the requisite accreditation standards, they are developing a culture of quality improvement that encourages administrators, faculty, and students to set goals and outcomes that extend far beyond meeting regulatory requirements. Instead, they are creating a teaching-learning environment in which reaching for excellence is exemplified throughout the program.

CONCLUSION

In many ways, the CQI Hallmark that states *"Program design, implementation, and evaluation are continuously reviewed and revised to achieve and maintain excellence"* can be thought of as the Hallmark that ultimately drives the achievement of excellence in the Hallmarks related to all the other categories. Whether faculty and administrators are focused on engaging students, developing faculty, designing curricula and teaching/learning strategies, acquiring resources, pursuing scholarship, or exhibiting institutional and professional leadership, they will not be successful in demonstrating excellence and achieving distinction in any of those areas, if they do not pursue those goals through the lens of CQI. An important first step for any faculty intent on maximizing program outcomes is to take the time to build an organizational culture that epitomizes the "Hallmarks" of an environment that has successfully instilled the values of CQI.

For these reasons, ensuring nursing administrators and faculty have opportunities to develop competence in quality assurance measures, program evaluation, and systems-thinking as applied to the educational environment is crucial for nursing programs to successfully navigate the complexities of higher education. When administrators, faculty, and staff are prepared to embrace the values of CQI and imbed them in their program planning and decision-making, the journey toward demonstrating excellence and achieving distinction in meeting program outcomes will be marked with success and recognized by all.

References

Boland, D. (2015). Program evaluation. In M. Oermann (Ed), *Teaching in nursing and role of the educator* (1st ed., pp. 275–299). Springer Publishing Company.

Eaton, J. S. (2012a). *Accreditation and recognition in the United States*. Council for Higher Education Accreditation. https://www.chea.org/overview-us-accreditation

Eaton, J. S. (2012b). *An overview of U.S. accreditation.* Council for Higher Education Accreditation. https://www.chea.org/overview-us-accreditation

Ellis, P. (2020). Systematic program evaluation. In D. Billings & J. Halstead (Ed.), *Teaching in nursing: A guide for faculty* (6th ed., pp. 514–559). Elsevier.

Ellis, P., & Halstead, J. (2012). Understanding the Commission on Collegiate Nursing Education accreditation process and the role of the continuous improvement progress report. *Journal of Professional Nursing, 28*(1), 18–26. https://doi:10.1016/j.profnurs.2011.10.004

Halstead, J. A. (2019). Program evaluation: Common challenges to data collection. *Teaching and Learning in Nursing, 14*(3), A6–A7. https://doi.org/10.1016/j.teln.2019.04.001

Halstead, J. A. (2020). Fostering innovation in nursing education: The role of accreditation. *Teaching and Learning in Nursing, 15*(1), A4–A5. https://doi.org/10.1016/j.teln.2019.10.003

National League for Nursing Commission for Nursing Education Accreditation. (2016). *Standards for accreditation*. https://cnea.nln.org/resources

Spector, N., Silvestri, J., Alexander, M., Martin, B., Hooper, J., Squires, A., & Ojemeni, M. (2020). NCSBN regulatory guidelines and evidence-based quality Indicators for nursing education programs. *Journal of Nursing Regulation, 11*(2; suppl.) S1–S64. https://www.ncsbn.org/Spector_NCSBN_Regulatory_Guidelines_and_Evidence_Based_Quality_Indicators_for_Nursing_education_programs.pdf

6

Achieving Excellence and Distinction in Nursing Education Through Innovative, Evidence-Based Curricula

Theresa M. "Terry" Valiga, EdD, RN, CNE, FAAN, ANEF

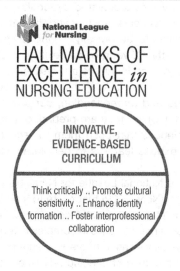

National League
for Nursing

HALLMARKS OF
EXCELLENCE *in*
NURSING EDUCATION

INNOVATIVE,
EVIDENCE-BASED
CURRICULUM

Think critically .. Promote cultural
sensitivity .. Enhance identity
formation .. Foster interprofessional
collaboration

INTRODUCTION

Oftentimes when faculty talk about "curriculum," they end up discussing specific courses, particular teaching strategies, or the best ways to evaluate student learning. In fact, two recent articles with the word "curriculum" in the title (Goncalves et al., 2020; Pagano et al., 2020) discussed particular teaching strategies rather than a curriculum, and while the strategies explained are exciting and of value to educators, they relate more to the learning process than to the overall curriculum.

While courses, teaching strategies, and evaluation methods are critical if students are to learn and grow professionally, it is important to keep in mind that they should not be addressed without consideration of the larger plan, which is known as the curriculum. Courses need to be developed within the context of overall goals that have been set by faculty; learning experiences need to be designed to ensure that students are enhancing their understanding of core concepts; and the overall approach to helping students grow and develop must progress in complexity, be logical, and make sense to all involved. It is these latter considerations that are key elements of the "curriculum" and that are discussed in this chapter.

One might think of the curriculum as the roadmap that allows one to arrive at a desired destination while having new and exciting experiences along the way. The route one chooses for the trip reflects certain values; for example, one might consider whether it is more important to arrive quickly or to visit friends/family and important historical sites along the way. The route must be planned carefully to avoid dead ends, unpaved roads, or lack of restrooms; however, it also should allow for some flexibility in case the journey presents some unexpected opportunities that are not to be missed. And the route should be plotted to provide opportunities for travelers to reflect on the towns and communities they visit, the people they meet, what they are learning, and how they are part of a larger context.

The curriculum designed to prepare students for new roles in nursing has similar components. It reflects the *values* articulated by faculty . . . what they believe about human beings, health and health care, society and the environment, nurses and nursing, and teaching/learning. It must be *logically organized* and *internally consistent* (i.e., make sense and "hang together"), yet provide *flexibility* that allows students to meet their individual learning needs and faculty to address issues and events that were not evident when the original plan was made. Finally, the curriculum should help students strengthen their *knowledge* and *understanding*, support them as they develop the *skills* needed for the role for which they are preparing, challenge students' *thinking*, engage students in experiences that push them to *reflect* on their own values and professional growth, and expose learners to people, ways of life, and perspectives that are *diverse*.

This chapter explores the National League for Nursing's (NLN's) *Hallmarks of Excellence in Nursing Education*© (NLN, 2020) that relate to innovative, evidence-based curricula. It explains and interrelates the essential components of a curriculum, addresses how core curriculum concepts need to build in complexity (from the beginning to the end of a particular program type, as well as from pre-licensure to master's to doctoral preparation), and explores the importance of ongoing refinement of the curriculum to ensure relevance.

ESSENTIAL COMPONENTS OF A CURRICULUM

One of the curriculum-related Hallmarks is that *the curriculum is designed to help students achieve stated program outcomes, reflects current societal and health care trends and issues, and is responsive to change and evolving societal needs.* This same Hallmark also notes that *the curriculum also embeds evidence-based information, reflects research findings and innovative practices, attends to the evolving role of the nurse in a variety of settings, is flexible and innovative, and incorporates local, national, and global perspectives.* To achieve this Hallmark, each key component of a curriculum needs serious discussion among faculty. Those components are as follows:

▸ Philosophy – Although many may be inclined to minimize the importance of this curriculum element, Valiga (2020) argues its significance and provides numerous examples of how the values articulated by faculty impact the development and implementation of the curriculum. One such example (p. 145) is that if the philosophical statement asserts a belief that "nurses must be prepared to provide leadership within their practice settings and for the profession as a whole," then one would expect to see "courses and learning experiences that help students appreciate the differences between leadership and management, study nursing leaders, and reflect on their own path toward becoming a leader."

▸ Conceptual or Overarching Framework – Faculty understand and appreciate the value and importance of a framework when designing a research study but often fail to realize its importance in curriculum work. Just as in research, the framework clearly identifies key concepts that will guide all that follows. For the curriculum, these key concepts help determine program outcomes, course foci, learning experiences, and evaluation measures, among other things.

▸ Design – Many nursing curricula today are designed to concentrate foundational learning in early semesters or years and concentrate learning experiences in nursing in later semesters/years. While there are benefits to this type of *building design*, curricula can be designed to provide for concurrent learning of nursing and foundational knowledge (i.e., *parallel design*) or reflect a *progressive design* that engages students in both areas of focus throughout the program but, over time, decreases the emphasis on foundational learning and increases the emphasis on nursing (Valiga, 2022).

▸ Implementation – This component of the curriculum focuses on specific course development, selection of strategies to facilitate learning, and choosing methods to evaluate student learning, all of which are discussed in detail in Chapter 7. Also important for this component are the resources needed (see Chapter 8) to provide for learning experiences that challenge and engage learners (see Chapter 3).

▸ Evaluation – As discussed fully in Chapter 5, when, how, and by whom the curriculum is evaluated is critical to ensure it remains relevant to today's reality, will prepare students to succeed in and help shape an uncertain tomorrow, and continues to meet the needs of increasingly diverse student populations.

Faculty will need to determine what they expect students to know, be able to do, and value upon graduation and articulate those program outcomes clearly. Thus, the curriculum must be designed to facilitate student growth in all three domains of learning: cognitive, psychomotor, and affective.

Faculty will need to determine the path students will take in relation to the key curriculum concepts selected (e.g., care management, collaboration, leadership, scholarship, professional identity). One path is the more traditional approach that organizes learning around specialty areas of practice (e.g., pediatrics, geriatrics, community health); another path follows a more concept-based approach (Giddens, 2020; Giddens & Brady, 2007) that organizes learning around practice-related concepts (e.g., oxygenation, mobility, professionalism); and yet another path is that of a competency-based approach (Lucey, 2018) that organizes learning to ensure that students achieve a predetermined level of performance in relation to a skill or area of knowledge before moving on to another skill or area of knowledge. A recent analysis of faculty experiences moving from a traditional to a concept-based curriculum (Wilhelm et al., 2020) provides insights about the differences in approach and things to consider when choosing among them.

In addition to attending to program outcomes, key curriculum concepts, and overall curriculum design or approach, faculty also would do well to consider the following Indicators related to this Hallmark:

> What opportunities are available for students to take courses in a sequence that makes sense to them or allows them to pursue study in areas in which they have learning needs?

> To what extent is the curriculum offered in flexible formats (e.g., part-time/full-time, day/evening, online/face-to-face/hybrid) to meet the individualized needs of students?

> What opportunities exist for students to participate in collaborative interprofessional practice?

> To what extent are students exposed to the role of the nurse in nontraditional, as well as traditional, settings?

> What opportunities exist for students to take electives or to choose course assignments or activities that match their interests and individual learning goals?

> To what extent can faculty members, students, and alumni identify the features of the program that are truly innovative and serve to distinguish it from other programs?

After careful consideration of these and other questions, faculty need to determine how they will help students advance from novices – who know nothing or very little about the new role for which they are preparing – to competent or even proficient (Benner, 1984) nurses. In other words, the curriculum must be developed to build in complexity and continually challenge learners to achieve deeper understandings, think more critically, perform skills more efficiently, and strengthen their identities as nurses and human beings.

CURRICULUM COMPLEXITY TO PREPARE FOR ROLE COMPLEXITY

The overarching goal of any nursing program is to prepare graduates to function effectively in the role they choose to pursue such as beginning clinician, advanced practice nurse, nurse educator, nurse administrator or executive, nurse scientist, and so on. Since each of these roles is complex and multifaceted, and since the individuals who implement these roles will be practicing in a world that is increasingly complex, ambiguous, technology-infused, ever-changing, and uncertain, the academic programs preparing them must also be complex and carefully designed. Indeed, "an enduring lesson of [the 2020] pandemic is that we do not know the future of the world for which we are preparing our students" (Matthews, 2020, p. 21).

As specified in the Hallmarks, the curriculum should *provide learning activities that enhance students' abilities to think critically, reflect thoughtfully, and provide culturally sensitive, evidence-based nursing care to diverse populations.* It also should *emphasize students' values development, identity formation, caring for self, commitment to lifelong learning, ethical and evidence-based practice, and creativity.* Clearly, such outcomes cannot be accomplished easily or all at once; thus, the curriculum needs to provide a logical route for students to build such abilities and enhance such insights.

To determine the path to success, curricula must be designed to help students achieve the stated program outcomes, outcomes that arise from the institution's mission, values of the profession, values expressed by faculty (as previously noted), the current and anticipated responsibilities and expectations of the role, external requirements and standards, and available resources. Since these outcomes are achieved only because of the many learning experiences students have from the beginning of a program to its end, they also are complex and multifaceted. In other words, program outcomes cannot be achieved in a single course, a single clinical experience, or completion of a dissertation or scholarly capstone project; the curriculum, therefore, needs to be designed to build in complexity and increasingly challenge learners as they progress through the program.

If faculty value tenets expressed by John Dewey (1899) regarding the importance of student-centered learning where the students' natural curiosity guides their exploration of ideas, they will design a curriculum that leads students to explore ideas of interest, learn more about themselves as learners and evolving professionals, and be fully engaged in the learning process. Such a curriculum may challenge learners to explore the need to attend to culture, race, socioeconomic status, and access to resources when planning and providing care to individual patients. That curriculum might then progress to challenging students to explore the factors that are critical when working as part of a team to provide care to a specific population or geographic community. And in its final phases, the curriculum might challenge students to propose strategies to influence policies related to access to care for vulnerable populations and reflect on the leadership skills they need to implement such strategies. If faculty agree that school plants "the seed of curiosity" (Westover, 2018, p. 60), they will design a curriculum that allows students' curiosity to flourish.

Another group of faculty might be in an institution that values service-learning, experiences designed to expose students to diverse populations and appreciate the contributions nurses can make as they collaborate with members of those populations to improve their health and their health care. In this case, students might first be expected to identify the challenges faced by members of the population that do or can have an impact on their health and well-being. As they advance through the program, students might be expected to meet with members of the community to identify priorities related to improving health and collaborate with them to propose strategies to address one or more of those priorities. Toward the end of the program, students might be expected to actively engage with key members of the population of interest and community leaders to implement and evaluate the impact of those strategies. Tillman et al. (2020) described how a service-learning experience in a military-sponsored free clinic served to positively impact the attitudes toward poverty and the underserved of students from six health profession programs. Nursing students expressed less bias toward and a decrease in stereotyping of the individuals served, and they expressed an increased willingness to advocate on behalf of those individuals when needed.

Faculty in another institution might design curricula to, among other goals, encourage and enhance deep learning. To achieve such a goal, learning experiences are deliberately designed to provide a foundation of knowledge, then to challenge students to critique that knowledge and use it to solve problems and formulate new ideas, and finally to construct a mental framework that allows the student to accept that more than one correct answer may exist, there is much that we do not know, and many perspectives may have validity. Wittmann-Price and Godshall (2009) described the use of a deep learning approach in clinical nursing courses and reported that it stimulated lifelong learning, improved students' critical thinking skills, enhanced conceptual learning (a finding also reported by Nielsen, 2016), promoted collaboration when attempting to solve problems, and enhanced students' abilities to transfer learning and insights gained from one context to another.

Considering their commitment to developing innovators and change agents/leaders who could drive improvement in health care, faculty in one university designed a curriculum with that goal in mind. Cusson et al. (2020) described how their curriculum helped undergraduate students prepare to take on the challenges of such roles. The Health Care Innovation Program (HCIP) they developed focused on "educating future registered nurses on the knowledge, skills, and attitudes required in order to identify problems, form scalable creative ideas, and subsequently begin developing those innovations to address health care needs of their patients, families, communities and populations in which they serve" (p. 14). After students were introduced to the concepts of innovation and change, they explored ways in which changes in practice might improve care, and concluded with a culminating experience that required them to work collaboratively to identify a clinical problem in need of an innovative solution (e.g., a product, process, or service), engage with key stakeholders to validate the identified problem, formulate a business plan to implement the innovation, and "pitch" their plan to stakeholders as well as faculty and student colleagues. Helping students achieve program outcomes related to leadership is a complex activity that must be planned carefully over a period of time and, therefore, calls for careful and deliberate curriculum planning.

Another example of how concepts can be addressed with increasing levels of complexity relates to what is likely to be a core curriculum concept, that of collaboration, both intra- and interprofessional. Students need first to develop their communication skills and understanding of the perspectives of individuals with varied roles and responsibilities in nursing (e.g., the unit manager or preceptor, the staff development educator or the clinical instructor) and those of other health professionals (e.g., physician, pharmacist, physical therapist). Such understandings could be achieved through a study of the preparation needed for each role, the current issues related to it, the challenges being faced by individuals in that role, licensure and/or certification requirements (if appropriate), and other factors. As students progress through their program, the curriculum design engages them in learning experiences where they need to collaborate with others – student peers, nurses on a clinical unit, members of a research team – to address problems of concern to all; such collaboration will help them sharpen communication skills and, quite likely, develop skills related to managing conflict. Final learning experiences could be designed to help students take the lead in collaborative efforts. The value of students from various health professions learning together – about each other and about the collaboration needed to provide quality care to diverse populations – was documented by Sigmon et al. (2020), who stated that participants in their study of nursing and medical students reported an appreciation for the contributions of all members of the healthcare team and a realization that when care was shared among professionals, patient satisfaction increased.

One additional example of deliberate curriculum design is the immersion clinical model, where baccalaureate students enrolled in nursing courses beginning in their freshman year participated in observational or limited field experiences during the first three years of study, then concentrated clinical learning experiences in the final year of study (Diefenbeck et al., 2006). Such a model reflects the beliefs of faculty that foundational knowledge and skills are essential prior to students' taking responsibility for the care of patients, and that "short" (i.e., four- or six-hour blocks of time) or interrupted (e.g., Tuesday and Thursday or only once per week) clinical experiences do not enhance students' confidence, do not allow them to truly be part of the healthcare team, and do not provide opportunities for them to identify care challenges and propose processes that can improve care. Outcomes of this curriculum model as reported by Diefenbeck et al. (2006) included the following: increased student confidence; enhanced relationships between students and staff, as well as between the school and the clinical agencies; less time spent "orienting" students and faculty to the setting; a more evident sense of "team"; the opportunity for students to delegate to assistive personnel; and the ability of faculty to teach slightly larger clinical groups.

One final example of how an internally consistent curriculum can be designed to enable students to meet program outcomes is that of the accelerated baccalaureate (ABSN) nursing program at the Duke University School of Nursing (https://nursing.duke.edu/academic-programs/absn-accelerated-bachelor-science-nursing/absn-curriculum). One of the key concepts in this curriculum is that of identity formation, which includes development of a sense of self as a professional nurse, a scholar, and a leader; attention to one's values, biases, and stereotypes; and internalization of the values of the profession. To help students achieve the program outcome related to this concept, the curriculum includes a course in each of the four semesters of the program that addresses Professional Nursing. In the first semester, the focus of this course is on "Past and Present"; the second-semester course addresses "Evolution as an Evidence-based Clinician"; the focus of the third-semester course is on the students' "Evolution as an Effective Team Member"; and in the final semester, the Professional Nursing course assists students in their "Evolution as a Leader." One can see from this progression of courses that the plan to help students develop and internalize an identity as a professional nurse, scholar, and leader is deliberate, and the material addressed in each becomes more complex and considers a broader sphere of involvement and influence.

The examples provided here illustrate how selected key curriculum concepts can be developed from the start to the end of a nursing education program: student-centered learning, service-learning, deep learning, development of innovators and change agents/leaders, intra- and interprofessional collaboration, immersion clinicals, and professional identity formation. As noted in the Hallmarks, however, there are many other concepts to be considered for deliberate development throughout a curriculum including care management, critical thinking, cultural sensitivity, evidence-based care, ethics, determinants of health, self-care, scholarship, information management, and others. Concepts can develop in complexity by moving from caring for patients with common health problems to caring for those with multisystem problems . . . from a focus on the individual to focusing on the family then the community and then populations . . . from attending to self-growth to enhancing the growth of others . . . from focusing on wellness to focusing on illness . . . from encompassing a narrow perspective to taking into consideration a broader, system-wide one . . . or along many other dimensions; the paths chosen will be influenced by the mission of the institution, faculty values, and a variety of external forces.

Finally, in addition to progressive and increasingly complex learning as previously described, it is important to keep in mind that there needs to be a logical progression from one program level to another (e.g., associate degree to baccalaureate [BSN], BSN to master's, BSN to DNP or PhD, master's to DNP or PhD) to ensure that expectations are higher, the scope of concern is broader, and skills related to the new role are developed. Several years ago, the NLN (2010) published a booklet that identified four key concepts – nursing judgment, human flourishing, professional identity, and spirit of inquiry – that have relevance for all program levels and, for each concept, suggested outcomes for each type of program. The ways in which outcomes increase in complexity across program type can serve as examples of goals toward which faculty would design curricula and specific learning experiences for students.

ONGOING REFINEMENT OF THE CURRICULUM

Curriculum development or revision is a lengthy, complex, and often exhausting process; once completed, faculty often are inclined to "leave it alone" for quite some time. When this occurs, curricula are likely to become outdated, fail to address concepts that are critical to the changing role of the nurse, and fail to engage students in learning experiences that prepare them to work with increasingly diverse populations who have challenging health needs and require new approaches to address those needs. Such outcomes will be avoided, however, when faculty develop and follow a total systematic program evaluation plan that guides them to regularly review the curriculum and refine or revise it as needed. In fact, one of the Hallmarks in this area notes that the curriculum must *reflect current societal healthcare trends and issues, be responsive to change and evolving societal needs, reflect research findings and innovative practices, and attend to the evolving role of the nurse in a variety of settings*. Thus, "curriculum work" never really is done.

One of the Indicators related to the curriculum Hallmarks asks faculty to reflect on the ways in which the curriculum is *regularly reviewed – with input from faculty members, students, and external stakeholders – and refined/revised as needed to incorporate current societal and health care trends and issues, research findings, innovative practices, and local as well as national and global perspectives.* Clearly, this work must involve all faculty, administrators, clinical partners, other key stakeholders, and the students who actually "live" the curriculum. The in-depth discussion of processes related to continuous quality improvement, including those related to the curriculum, offered in Chapter 5 will be helpful to faculty in their efforts to design and implement innovative, evidence-based curricula and ultimately achieve excellence in their educational programs and distinction for their school/institution.

Faculty also would do well to read Al-Alawi and Alexander's (2020) systematic review of program evaluation in nursing programs. Although this review focused on baccalaureate programs, the findings have relevance for post-baccalaureate/graduate programs as well. These authors noted that the most common variables evaluated to determine program effectiveness were student satisfaction, students' perceptions of their learning experiences, and stakeholders' (e.g., alumni, employers, and faculty) perceptions of program quality and graduate competencies. They also concluded that most data related to program effectiveness were summative in nature and collected upon program completion; however, they also issued the following ideas for serious consideration: "In the context of a growing body of literature suggesting the importance of formative evaluation in generating continuous improvement in program implementation and ensuring efficiency in channeling budgets, human resources, and time in a productive manner . . . examining program inputs, processes, and activities throughout program delivery is just as important as examining program outcomes" (p. 241).

Perhaps the even more critical step in curriculum evaluation efforts, however, is that of *using* data that are collected to ensure the curriculum meets accreditation standards (Commission on Collegiate Nursing Education [CCNE], 2018; NLN Commission on Nursing Education Accreditation [CNEA], 2016), is responsive to recommendations from professional groups such as the Interprofessional Education Collaborative Expert Panel (2011), and attends to the recently distributed Regulatory Guidelines and Evidence-based Quality Indicators for Nursing Education Programs (National Council of State Boards of Nursing [NCSBN], 2020) and other key resources. In his book of mistakes, Prichard (2018) stated that "mediocrity is the end result of too much comfort. All growth requires discomfort" (p. 100). Those schools/institutions that choose to pursue excellence in nursing education and wish to distinguish themselves from other schools/institutions will also challenge themselves to achieve the Hallmarks related to the curriculum and use the "discomfort" associated with that growth to design, implement, continually evaluate, and revise as needed relevant, internally consistent, engaging, innovative, and evidence-based curricula for all students.

CONCLUSION

There is no question that curriculum work is difficult and challenging. But it must be done in a deliberate way if students are to engage in learning experiences that make sense, grow in complexity, and effectively prepare them for the beginning or advanced nursing role they wish to implement.

Faculty are challenged to ensure that the curriculum is relevant and responsive, a fact that has become all too clear in light of the 2020 COVID-19 pandemic. This experience should be a "wake-up call" for all nursing programs to reflect on what it is students truly need to know, do, and value as the result of engaging in a particular academic program.

Some may think that the pandemic leads to a conclusion that we need to add more content on communicable diseases; this suggestion certainly has merit, but we must be careful not to create an even more overloaded curriculum. It seems, however, we also may need to pay more attention to how we help students deal with fear, uncertainty, conflicting information, and the raw emotions of those experiencing health crises. We may need to consider how we help students attend to their own physical and mental health and well-being while caring for others, as well as how we help them appreciate and respond to the needs of colleagues on the healthcare team.

The pandemic experience challenges faculty to think about how they help students find, judge, and use (or not use) information that is relevant to the safe, quality care of their patients, their colleagues, and themselves. It has made us think about the emphasis we do or do not place on population health, prevention strategies, access to care, healthcare policy, and the leadership skills needed by nurses to advocate for the underserved and vulnerable.

As stated by Morin (2020, p. 3118), "perhaps the time is now to reconsider what constitutes critical information and competencies," and although she addressed this specifically to pre-licensure programs, it is just as relevant to master's, DNP, and PhD programs. Morin also presented the challenge that "it is time to move from a focus on content to a focus on competency-based education" (p. 3118) and cited evidence from neuroscience of teaching and learning to suggest that "distributing disciplinary content over all years of the curriculum [rather than concentrating it in the final two years] may provide students the opportunity and time to process and practice what they are learning" (p. 3118).

It is hoped that faculty who make thoughtful decisions about how best to prepare students for complex nursing roles and design curricula that reflect the Hallmarks discussed here will graduate individuals who have the knowledge/understanding, skills, and values that allow them to function as excellent clinicians, midwives, clinical nurse specialists, nurse practitioners, educators, administrators/executives, informaticists, and scientists who will shape the future of our profession and health care. Such is the power of continually striving for excellence and aiming to achieve distinction in nursing education.

References

Al-Alawi, R., & Alexander, G. L. (2020). Systematic review of program evaluation in baccalaureate nursing programs. *Journal of Professional Nursing, 36*(4), 236–244. https://doi.org/10.1016/j.profnurs.2019.12.003

Benner, P. (1984). *From novice to expert*. Prentice-Hall.

Commission on Collegiate Nursing Education. (2018). *Standards for accreditation of baccalaureate and graduate nursing programs (Amended)*. Author. https://www.aacnnursing.org/Portals/42/CCNE/PDF/Standards-Final-2018.pdf

Cusson, R. M., Meehan, C., Bourgault, A., & Kelley, T. (2020). Educating the next generation of nurses to be innovators and change agents. *Journal of Professional Nursing, 36*, 13–19. https://doi.org/10.1016/j.profnurs.2019.07.004

Dewey, J. (1899). *School and society*. University of Chicago Press.

Diefenbeck, C., Plowfield, L., & Herrman, J. (2006). Clinical immersion: A residency model for nursing education. *Nursing Education Perspectives, 27*(2), 71–79. https://doi.org/10.3928/01484834-20200220-01

Giddens, J. (2020). Demystifying concept-based and competency-based approaches (Guest Editorial). *Journal of Nursing Education, 59*(3), 123–124. https://doi.org/10.3928/01484834-20200220-01

Giddens, J., & Brady, D. P. (2007). Rescuing nursing education from content saturation: The case for a concept-based curriculum. *Journal of Nursing Education, 46*(2), 65–69. https://doi.org/10.3928/01484834-20070201-05

Goncalves, S. A., Treas, L. S., & Wilkinson, J. M. (2020). Bringing caring back into the curriculum through innovative iCare feature. *Nursing Education Perspectives, 41*(6), 381–382. https://doi.org/10.1097/01.NEP.0000000000000525

Interprofessional Education Collaborative Expert Panel. (2011). *Core competencies for interprofessional collaborative practice: Report of an Expert Panel*. Author. https://www.aacom.org/docs/default-source/insideome/ccrpt05-10-11.pdf?sfvrsn=77937f97_2

Lucey, C. R. (2018). *Achieving competency-based, time-variable health professions education. Proceedings of a conference sponsored by Josiah Macy Jr. Foundation in June 2017*. Josiah Macy Jr. Foundation. https://macyfoundation.org/assets/reports/publications/macy_monograph_2017_final.pdf

Matthews, K. (2020). Revisiting John Dewey's message about community. *Phi Kappa Phi Forum, 100*(4), 21.

Morin, K. H. (2020). Nursing education after COVID-19: Same or different? (Editorial). *Journal of Clinical Nursing, 29*(17-18), 3117–3119. https://doi.org/10.1111/jocn.15322

National Council of State Boards of Nursing. (2020). NCSBN regulatory guidelines and evidence-based quality Indicators for nursing education programs. *Journal of Nursing Regulation, 11*(2, supplement), entire issue. https://www.ncsbn.org/Spector_NCSBN_Regulatory_Guidelines_and_Evidence_Based_Quality_Indicators_for_Nursing_education_programs.pdf

National League for Nursing. (2010). *Outcomes and competencies for graduates of practical/vocational, diploma, associate degree, baccalaureate, master's, practice doctorate, and research doctorate programs in nursing*. Author.

National League for Nursing. (2020). *Hallmarks of excellence in nursing education*. Author. http://www.nln.org/professional-development-programs/teaching-resources/hallmarks-of-excellence

National League for Nursing Commission on Nursing Education Accreditation. (2016). *Accreditation standards for nursing education programs*. Author.

http://www.nln.org/docs/default-source/accreditation-services/cnea-standards-final-february-201613f2bf5c78366c709642ff00005f0421.pdf?sfvrsn=12&_ga=2.118230857.1381909281.1611323886-1992668941.1557668811

Nielsen, A. (2016). Concept-based learning in clinical experiences: Bringing theory to clinical education for deep learning. *Journal of Nursing Education, 55*(7), 365–371. https://doi.org/10.3928/01484834-20160615-02

Pagano, M., Mager, D. R., O'Shea, E. R., & O'Sullivan, C. (2020). Evaluation of an innovative curriculum enhancement: The conversation project. *Nursing Education Perspectives, 41*(6), 382–383. https://doi.org/10.1097/01.NEP.0000000000000541

Prichard, S. (2018). *The book of mistakes: 9 secrets to creating a successful future*. Hachett Book Group.

Sigmon, L. B., Woodard, E. K., & Woody, G. (2020). Quality Olympics: Experiential interprofessional learning to improve quality and safety. *Journal of Nursing Education, 59*(10), 589–593. https://doi.org/10.3928/01484834-20200921-10

Tillman, P., Thomas, M., & Buelow, J. R. (2020). Impact of service learning on student attitudes toward the poor and underserved. *Nurse Educator, 45*(6), 316–319. https://doi.org/10.1097/NNE.0000000000000807

Valiga, T. M. (2020). Philosophical foundations of the curriculum. In D. M. Billings & J. A. Halstead, *Teaching in nursing: A guide for faculty* (6th ed., pp. 135–146). Elsevier.

Valiga, T. M. (2022). Curriculum models and course development. In M. H. Oermann, J. C. De Gagne, & B. C. Phillips (Eds.), *Teaching in nursing and role of the educator: The complete guide to best practice in teaching, evaluation, and curriculum development* (3rd ed., pp. 343–355). Springer.

Westover, T. (2018). *Educated: A memoir*. Random House.

Wilhelm, S., Rodehorst, T. K., & Longoria, A. (2020). Transitioning from a traditional to a concept-based curriculum: Faculty's experience. *Nursing Education Perspectives*, *41*(6), 355–357. https://doi.org/10.1097/01.NEP.0000000000000562

Wittmann-Price, R. A., & Godshall, M. (2009). Strategies to promote deep learning in clinical nursing courses. *Nurse Educator*, *34*(5), 214–216. https://doi.org/10.1097/NNE.0b013e3181b2b576

7

Achieving Excellence and Distinction Through the Use of Innovative, Evidence-Based Approaches to Facilitate and Evaluate Learning

Marilyn H. Oermann, PhD, RN, FAAN, ANEF

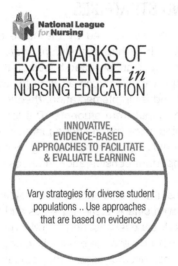

National League *for* **Nursing**

HALLMARKS OF
EXCELLENCE *in*
NURSING EDUCATION

INNOVATIVE,
EVIDENCE-BASED
APPROACHES TO FACILITATE
& EVALUATE LEARNING

Vary strategies for diverse student
populations .. Use approaches
that are based on evidence

INTRODUCTION

Teaching in nursing is an interpersonal process: teachers interact with students in a wide range of learning environments with the goal of facilitating learning. In some learning environments, this interaction is direct—teachers and students learn together in classrooms, simulations, and clinical settings. In other environments such as in online courses, interactions between teachers and students still occur, but may be asynchronous and developed through discussions and learning activities in which students engage with their peers and the educator virtually, rather than face-to-face. Regardless of the environment, the teacher's ability and willingness to actively involve students are critical in promoting learning. Teaching is more than telling students the information they need to learn or demonstrating procedures and interventions; instead, good teaching engages students as active participants in the learning process.

Good teaching involves creating a learning environment in which students are comfortable with sharing ideas, raising questions, and exploring new ways of thinking. In such an environment, the teacher is viewed as a resource for students as they discover knowledge for themselves. This does not indicate a lack of goals or outcomes to be achieved; instead, teachers carefully design learning activities and select teaching strategies that will enable students to meet learning outcomes. Teachers also need to create the supportive environment in which students can learn.

The purpose of this chapter is to explore innovative and evidence-based teaching and evaluation strategies, propose guidelines for selecting these for nursing courses, and relate these efforts to the goal of achieving excellence in nursing education. The teaching and evaluation methods selected for discussion in the chapter demonstrate the wide range of evidence available to guide decisions about methods to use in nursing education.

SELECTING TEACHING STRATEGIES

Teaching strategies are methods planned by the nurse educator to guide student learning and development. In this chapter, the word *strategy* is used interchangeably with the word *method*. Strategies are selected based on the learning outcomes to be met, students' needs, other variables such as time for the instruction, evidence to support use of a method and its implementation, theories and concepts that guide learning and teaching, and input from students. The learning outcomes are key in selecting teaching strategies since the methods planned for a course and what students do in the course should align with the learning outcomes. Thus, the outcomes to be met are the most important consideration in choosing methods for teaching in a course.

The individual needs of students also should be considered. Nursing students are a diverse group of learners, with different learning styles and preferences, cultural backgrounds, ages, life and work experiences, and knowledge. Students will be impeded in their learning if they do not possess the prerequisite knowledge and skills. Through carefully designed questions, diagnostic quizzes, students' self-assessments, and other strategies, the teacher determines students' present level of understanding that would influence their achieving the outcomes. These gaps in understanding must be addressed first. By varying teaching strategies, the educator is more likely to meet the learning needs of the diverse group of students and meet the Hallmark of Excellence in Nursing Education© that states *Strategies used to facilitate and evaluate learning by a diverse student population are innovative and varied*.

Time for instruction is another consideration in selecting teaching strategies. Lecture, for example, may be the most efficient method to communicate specific information to students that they need for understanding patient conditions and typical care measures, essential to engage in problem solving and higher level thinking.

Some teaching strategies in nursing education, such as simulation, are well studied, and evidence is available to guide their use. Other strategies have limited research support, but they nevertheless reflect relevant theories of how students learn best and ways to promote their learning. In deciding on teaching and evaluation approaches to use in a course, educators should evaluate the evidence that is available on the strategy and its implementation. All too often nurse educators do not search for evidence on which to base their decisions. Some faculty use the same methods they experienced as students or the same approaches year after year without reflection as to better ways to guide student learning based on the current course outcomes and learner population.

Another Hallmark is that *Strategies to facilitate and evaluate learning used by faculty members are evidence-based*. Evidence-based teaching involves using the findings of research as a basis for decisions about teaching strategies, evaluation methods, and other educational practices used in a course (Oermann, 2018, 2020). Strong evidence is generated from well-designed and rigorous research studies that use validated measures. The quality of the research is critical in deciding whether to use a teaching or evaluation method and how best to implement it (Oermann, 2020). Similar to evidence-based practice, systematic reviews, in which multiple high-quality study findings are synthesized, provide the highest level of evidence, followed by randomized controlled trials, cohort studies, descriptive studies, and expert opinions (Oermann, 2022). In other words, a systematic review on a potential teaching method provides stronger evidence than a few descriptive studies carried out in one school of nursing.

In selecting teaching strategies, the nurse educator also considers learning theories, theories of motivation, readiness to learn, concepts of student engagement and active learning, and styles of learning, among others. Finally, the teacher's own philosophy of teaching and expertise also enter into decisions about educational approaches to use, and students should have input as to their preferences and own goals for learning (Oermann, 2022).

TEACHING STRATEGIES

Active Learning

The need for active learning is well established in the literature. With active learning, students "do something" in order to learn — they are engaged as active participants in the instruction. With many of these strategies, students work collaboratively to analyze cases, develop solutions to real-life problems, critique different approaches, and share varied perspectives, all of which reflects a constructivist approach to learning where students gain new knowledge and deepen understanding as a result of their own experiences. Courses can be designed to provide an environment for active learning such as with problem-based learning (PBL), team-based learning (TBL), and flipped classrooms. However, there are many teaching methods that involve active learning and can be used in a course: discussions of ideas with peers, group activities, case analyses, written assignments, projects, and other activities in which students need to think about the content and *use* it in new situations. Active learning also can be integrated in teaching methods in which students are typically more passive learners, for example, pausing lectures for students to work through related cases in small groups.

Many studies support active learning across fields and levels of students. In a large meta-analysis (a statistical method that combines the results of individual studies),

Freeman et al. (2014) examined 225 studies on student performance in undergraduate science, technology, engineering, and mathematics (STEM) courses comparing traditional lecture to active learning strategies. Student examination scores were higher in courses with active learning compared to lecture, a finding that was consistent across different types of courses, levels, and numbers of students in the course. However, active learning was most effective when classes were small (50 or fewer students). Although this study did not include nursing courses, it provides strong evidence of the outcomes of active learning for application to nursing education.

Another meta-analysis extended these findings and documented that underrepresented students taking STEM courses performed better on examinations in classes with active learning compared to traditional lectures (Theobald et al., 2020). Student examination scores from 15 studies (9,238 total students) and student failure rates from 26 studies (44,606 total students) were analyzed. The extent of time students engaged in active learning in class was important: the meta-analysis found that classes that implemented high-intensity active learning strategies were most effective. This study provides strong evidence to support teaching strategies that use active learning not only in STEM disciplines but also in other fields such as nursing.

Problem-Based Learning

In PBL, students work in groups to identify and analyze problems, propose solutions, and learn to collaborate with others, including the teacher who often is a resource for the student groups rather than an answer-provider. In this process they gain knowledge; develop higher level cognitive skills such as problem solving, critical thinking, and clinical judgment; and learn to work in groups to solve problems and resolve conflicts (Carvalho et al., 2017; Y. Li et al., 2019; Sayyah et al., 2017; Wosinski et al., 2018). Studies not only support the outcomes of PBL but also have provided evidence on best practices when implementing this method in a course (Wosinski et al., 2018).

Team-Based Learning

TBL is an active learning strategy with three specific phases as part of the method. Students begin with pre-class preparation that often includes prerecorded lectures and readings; the goal of the pre-class assignments is to provide the knowledge base students need to engage in active learning and group activities in class. In the second phase, students take individual and group readiness assurance tests related to the content they learned in the pre-class assignments. The third phase consists of a group learning activity in which students apply the content to case scenarios and answer questions as a team (Michaelsen et al., 2008). Additional learning occurs as teams present to the entire class their decisions and how they reached them. While TBL is student-centered, the role of faculty is to ask questions to extend learning and reinforce key concepts, as well as to facilitate the strategy and provide feedback to students as they are learning in teams (Koh et al., 2020).

Systematic reviews support TBL as an effective teaching strategy in health professions education. Most of the research has found that TBL improves academic performance, promotes student engagement, and involves active learning (Dearnley et al.,

2018; Fatmi et al., 2013; Reimschisel et al., 2017; Sisk, 2011). In the review by Reimschisel et al. of 118 studies on TBL in health professions education, 85 examined the outcomes of TBL; of these, 61 percent concluded that TBL improved learning and was an effective technique. Student satisfaction with TBL has been mixed, but in Reimschisel et al.'s review, students reported that they preferred TBL to more traditional teaching methods such as lecture. Positive features of TBL from the students' perspective were interactions with peers, active learning, and the opportunity to apply content they were learning to cases and discuss the content with others. Dearnley et al. (2018) reviewed 16 studies on TBL in nursing and concluded that TBL had an impact on student engagement, satisfaction, academic performance, and transformative learning, but more research was needed.

Flipped Classroom

Flipped classrooms share many of the attributes of TBL such as pre-class preparation and in-class collaborative work with peers on problem-solving exercises, analyses of cases, and other small group activities. Evidence on the outcomes of flipped classrooms in nursing education, however, has been mixed. In a review by Ward et al. (2018) of 14 studies on flipped classrooms, most students reported that the in-class activities were valuable and provided interaction and engagement in learning. Only five studies measured learning outcomes when the flipped classroom was used; four of these studies reported that flipped classes had a positive impact on student grades. Students' preferences regarding traditional or flipped classrooms were mixed. Evans et al. (2019) conducted a systematic review of 24 studies; eight studies found no significant differences in academic performance between flipped classrooms and traditional teaching methods. In four studies, posttest scores were higher than pretest, but it was not clear if the change was due to the flipped teaching method. These researchers concluded that there was no compelling evidence of the effectiveness of flipped classes above traditional classroom approaches.

In a meta-analysis of 11 randomized controlled trials, Hu et al. (2018) found that students' theoretical knowledge and skill scores were significantly higher in a flipped classroom compared to traditional lectures ($p < .001$). In another systematic review and meta-analysis of 22 studies of Chinese nursing students, the researchers reported similar findings: flipped classrooms compared to traditional lecture improved skill competence scores, cooperation and sense of teamwork among students, communication, interest in participating in the course, ability to think about and analyze problems, and satisfaction with the course, among other outcomes (Xu et al., 2019). However, these researchers, consistent with others, concluded that larger samples and higher quality studies were needed to strengthen the evidence on flipped classrooms.

Small Group Learning

Small group learning includes any strategy in which students work in small groups to solve problems, work through clinical cases, and complete other learning activities with peers. With this method, students work collaboratively to gain new knowledge about the content, develop their problem-solving and critical thinking skills, and learn from each other. Strategies in which students work in small groups in class, in an online environment, and in other formats are student-centered, providing for active learning.

A meta-analysis on the effectiveness of different types of small group learning methods on student achievement revealed that these methods improved students' academic achievement in nursing and other health science classes (Kalaian & Kasim, 2017). These authors analyzed 19 studies with 4,050 students, 1,560 of whom were in nursing and other health science courses that used small group methods, and the remaining 2,490 were in courses with lecture-based instruction. Seventeen of the 19 studies reviewed indicated that small group learning was more effective than lecture in increasing scores on standardized and teacher-developed examinations.

Questions

Asking open-ended and thought-provoking questions is an effective strategy for promoting students' higher-level thinking. Through questions, students can share their thinking and the process they used to arrive at decisions or judgments. Questions also are an effective strategy for assessing students' knowledge and understanding of concepts, as well as their ability to apply learning to new situations. The level of questions guides the interaction toward the learning outcomes and, more importantly, determines the level of thinking required by students. Questions can be low-level, focusing on recalling facts and specific information; however, while this level of question assesses if students have the requisite knowledge for engaging in critical thinking and making judgments about a clinical situation, in most learning situations the goal is to foster higher level thinking (Oermann & Gaberson, 2021; Oermann et al., 2018). Asking students questions to explore their understanding, make connections across concepts, probe assumptions and reasoning, consider multiple perspectives, and reflect on their own thinking can improve students' critical thinking (Dinkins & Cangelosi, 2019; Hagler & Morris, 2022; Makhene, 2019; Oermann & Gaberson, 2021).

Some studies have suggested that while nurse educators strive to ask higher level questions, many of the questions tend to be at the recall and lower levels of thinking. In a scoping review of 19 studies, Merisier et al. (2018) found that nurse educators asked mainly low-level questions that frequently required only a yes or no answer, findings that are consistent with earlier studies (Phillips & Duke, 2001; Phillips et al., 2017; Profetto-McGrath et al., 2004). Awareness of the tendency to ask recall and closed-ended questions and an opportunity to practice asking higher level questions may be effective for educators to raise the level of their questions. In a study by Phillips et al. (2017), most of the questions asked by 133 clinical nurse educators and preceptors were at the knowledge level and required only recalling facts. However, participants who had taken an education-related workshop or course asked significantly more questions at higher cognitive levels, leading the authors to recommend that educators could benefit from targeted instruction on how to frame questions that stimulate application and analytical thinking.

Cases

Cases provide a clinical scenario or describe another type of situation for students to analyze. Typically, the scenario presents new information for students to apply their knowledge from class, to interpret, and to make decisions. Cases engage students in thinking through patient problems they may not have encountered in clinical practice, analyzing data and deciding on additional data to collect, identifying possible problems, weighing alternative actions, and making decisions and learning from them (Cleveland et al., 2015; Hong & Yu, 2017; S. Li et al., 2019; Oermann & Gaberson, 2021; Thistleth-waite et al., 2012; Vacek & Liesveld, 2020). Although cases can be completed individually, they can be particularly effective for small group analysis where students can critique each other's thinking about the scenario and compare different interpretations and approaches to addressing the problem at hand (Oermann & Gaberson, 2021).

Cases have two parts: a situation (scenario) and open-ended questions about it (see Box 7-1 for examples of scenarios and questions). One scenario can be used, or it can unfold with new data added that might change the analysis and decisions. The scenarios can integrate knowledge from across units or modules in a course, across courses in the curriculum, or from non-nursing foundational courses as well as nursing ones; ethical situations for students to recognize and think about best responses; and quality and safety outcomes, among others. The questions asked about the scenario are key to the effectiveness of this strategy, and typically open-ended questions with more than one correct answer will lead to higher level thinking and discussions.

BOX 7-1

Sample Cases

Sample Case 1

Your patient is admitted for a cardiac catheterization. In your assessment, he tells you he has a head-ache and feels dizzy, but it "might be from not eating breakfast." His vital signs are temperature 37.4°C, pulse 106 bpm, respirations 22 per minute, and blood pressure 178/90.
1. What findings are most significant?
2. What additional information is needed?
3. What questions would you ask him next? Why is this information important?

Sample Case 2

A mother brings her 2-month-old infant to the public health department for a check-up. She tells you that she is having "trouble feeding the baby." The infant is whimpering but has no tears and seems restless. You take the infant's weight, and it is 8 lbs. 5 oz.
1. What are possible problems with this infant? Provide a rationale for each of the problems you are considering.
2. What other assessment data would you expect to find?
3. What additional information do you need as a priority to support your findings?

Sample Case 3

A patient returns to the long-term care setting after having an ultrasound and a CT scan. The patient's vital signs are temperature 38.5°C, pulse 130 bpm, respirations 24 per min, and blood pressure 90/60. The patient tells the nursing assistant he "feels lousy." There is nothing documented when the patient voided last or had a meal.
1. What concerns you in this scenario? Discuss in your small group.
2. What are all possible problems of this patient?
3. Discuss what the nurse should do next.

An early review of evidence indicated that cases were enjoyable to do, students perceived they learned from cases, and faculty supported cases for active learning (Thistlethwaite et al., 2012). However, the findings were inconclusive as to the impact of cases on learning outcomes. More recent studies suggest cases may improve critical thinking and depth of learning, enhance clinical knowledge, improve group interactions, and promote clinical reasoning (S. Li et al., 2019; McLean, 2016; Wosinski et al., 2018).

Lecture

Lecture has been a predominant teaching strategy in nursing education and other fields. With the focus on active learning, many faculty have shifted away from lecture to active learning and small group activities based on strong evidence supporting these strategies. However, some outcomes and content areas may be best taught with a lecture. Lecture provides an effective method of communicating specific information to students. In a lecture the teacher can integrate key content from various sources and research findings, explain difficult concepts to students, and provide examples of application to clinical practice. Gooblar (2019) suggested that lectures should be supplemented with learning activities in which students *use* the information in some way and identify gaps in their own knowledge.

Implementation of New Teaching Strategies

As nurse educators consider various teaching strategies for their courses, it is important to review the evidence supporting their potential uses and outcomes. Equally important is to understand the techniques of the method, guiding how it should be implemented. Studies have not been done in nursing education on how faculty adopt evidence in their teaching and successfully implement new strategies in their courses. Do faculty use educational innovations and teaching methods as designed, or do they modify them for their courses and to meet faculty and student needs? If they make modifications, does that affect learning outcomes, and if it does, what is that effect? Some teaching strategies such as TBL have specific phases and requirements as part of the pedagogy, but most teaching strategies — even those with a strong evidence base — allow more flexibility when adopting them for a course.

Cianciolo and Regehr (2019) suggested that teaching methods and educational innovations have three layers: techniques (how to use the method), related principles, and educational philosophy on which the method or innovation is based. These suggest areas of discussion for faculty prior to implementing a new method or approach, which is an approach consistent with another Hallmark: *Faculty members engage in collegial dialogue and interact with students and colleagues in nursing and other professions to promote and develop strategies to facilitate and evaluate learning.*

Faculty should understand the evidence (i.e., the research) that supports the method, the principles and theory that underlie it, and whether the method they are considering can be tailored to meet their local needs without influencing its effectiveness. An examination of barriers and facilitators to implementing educational evidence and innovations in a nursing program and course or of the processes that faculty use when adopting new methods have not been examined and, therefore, are areas in which further research is needed in nursing education.

EVALUATION STRATEGIES

In nursing courses, faculty not only need to make informed decisions about teaching strategies but also about methods for evaluating student learning outcomes. Evaluation is the process of making judgments about students' achievement of the course outcomes, quality of clinical performance, and other areas of learning (Oermann & Gaberson, 2021). Decisions about students' progress in meeting the learning outcomes and developing clinical competencies represent formative evaluation. This form of evaluation occurs throughout the learning process and provides feedback to students that guides them to fill gaps in their knowledge and competency (Brookhart & Nitko, 2019; Oermann & Gaberson, 2021). Summative evaluation determines if students met the outcomes and developed the expected clinical competencies; it leads to judgments about what has been learned and is the basis for determining grades in courses.

There are many evaluation methods for use in nursing courses. These methods include tests (teacher-made and standardized), written assignments, small group activities, presentations, group projects, and strategies used commonly in clinical courses such as observations of performance, rating scales, electronic portfolios, simulation-based assessments, and objective structured clinical examinations (OCSEs), among others. In some courses, the same evaluation methods are used year after year without consideration as to whether they are the best approaches for assessing the learning outcomes. The goal for educators is to select evaluation strategies to determine if students are making progress in meeting or have achieved the course outcomes and clinical competencies. The way in which faculty decide on evaluation methods for a course has not been studied, but these decisions can be guided by seven best practices summarized in Box 7-2.

Some evaluation strategies in nursing education, such as tests and OSCEs, are well studied, and evidence is available to support their use. Objective structured clinical examination, designed for evaluating the performance of a learner in a laboratory or simulation setting or via technology instead of in the clinical setting, is a good example of an evaluation method supported by research. In an OSCE, students rotate through stations where their performance is evaluated, usually by multiple examiners. At some stations, students may perform assessments, clinical skills, and procedures, while at other stations, they may analyze cases and plan care (Oermann & Gaberson, 2021). Some OSCEs include use of standardized patients. Studies on OSCEs indicate they provide a valid and reliable method for evaluating performance of varied skills and competencies (Goh et al., 2019; Selim & Dawood, 2015). Goh et al.'s systematic review of 204 studies in nursing education not only documented the validity and reliability of OSCEs, but this review also provided guidelines for how to use an OSCE for an evaluation.

Other evaluation methods such as written assignments have limited research support but are guided by best practices. For example, written assignments should build on one another in a course and across courses; they should not be repetitive; and if part of the goal of such an exercise is to help students develop their writing skills, submission of multiple drafts is valuable.

BOX 7-2

Guidelines for Selecting Evaluation Methods

1. Evaluation methods in a course should be selected based on the learning outcomes to be evaluated. Be clear about *what* to evaluate, then choose a method that provides the information needed to determine if students met the outcome.
2. Every evaluation method in a course should relate to at least one of the learning outcomes or it is not needed. Review the methods in your course to ensure they are relevant.
3. There should be a reasonable number of evaluation methods in a course. Many methods such as tests and written assignments collect information about multiple outcomes. By matching the evaluation method to an outcome, you can ensure an appropriate number of methods used in a course.
4. Varied evaluation methods should be used in a course rather than only one method such as tests. By varying the methods, you also reflect the diversity of students' learning styles and strengths.
5. Students need to know what is expected of them in a course. The relationship of the evaluation method to the course outcome(s) should be apparent.
6. Providing feedback to students is an important role of the nurse educator. The methods for evaluation should provide specific information about students' progress for the educator to share and use for further instruction.
7. Nurse educators should always consider the limitations of any evaluation method. There are many factors that can influence students' achievement on a test, on an assignment, and in clinical practice on a particular day. Judgments about a student's learning and performance should not be based on an evaluation done one time.

Adapted from Oermann, M., & Gaberson, K. (2021). *Evaluation and testing in nursing education* (6th ed.). Springer Publishing Company.

CONCLUSION

Teaching and evaluation strategies should be selected based on the learning outcomes to be met, evidence to support their use, and theories and concepts that guide learning and teaching, among other factors. The learning outcomes are key, so it is essential that the methods planned for a course align with the learning outcomes. For some methods evidence is available to guide decisions, and it is up to the nurse educator to search for and review this evidence. Other methods, however, have not been studied, and in those situations, it is up to the educator to have a clear understanding of theories and concepts of learning as a framework for decisions about educational approaches to use. Many decisions about teaching and evaluation are based on the educator's judgment about the best methods to use. These judgments should reflect an understanding of the method or educational approach guided by the nursing education and educational literature and discussions with colleagues: these are Hallmarks in nursing education.

References

Brookhart, S. M., & Nitko, A. J. (2019). *Educational assessment of students* (8th ed.). Pearson Education.

Carvalho, D., Azevedo, I. C., Cruz, G. K. P., Mafra, G. A. C., Rego, A. L. C., Vitor, A. F., Santos, V. E. P., Cogo, A. L. P., & Ferreira Júnior, M. A. (2017). Strategies used for the promotion of critical thinking in nursing undergraduate education: A systematic review. *Nurse Education Today, 57*, 103–107. https://doi.org/10.1016/j.nedt.2017.07.010

Cianciolo, A. T., & Regehr, G. (2019). Learning theory and educational intervention: Producing meaningful evidence of impact through layered analysis. *Academic Medicine, 94*(6), 789–794. https://doi.org/10.1097/acm.0000000000002591

Cleveland, L. M., Carmona, E. V., Paper, B., Solis, L., & Taylor, B. (2015). Baby Boy Jones interactive case-based learning activity: A web-delivered teaching strategy. *Nurse Educator, 40*(4), 179–182. https://doi.org/10.1097/nne.0000000000000129

Dearnley, C., Rhodes, C., Roberts, P., Williams, P., & Prenton, S. (2018). Team based learning in nursing and midwifery higher education; a systematic review of the evidence for change. *Nurse Education Today, 60*, 75–83. https://doi.org/10.1016/j.nedt.2017.09.012

Dinkins, C., & Cangelosi, P. (2019). Putting Socrates back in Socratic method: Theory-based debriefing in the nursing classroom. *Nursing Philosophy, 20*(2), e12240. https://doi.org/10.1111/nup.12240

Evans, L., Vanden Bosch, M. L., Harrington, S., Schoofs, N., & Coviak, C. (2019). Flipping the classroom in health care higher education: A systematic review. *Nurse Educator, 44*(2), 74–78. https://doi.org/10.1097/nne.0000000000000554

Fatmi, M., Hartling, L., Hillier, T., Campbell, S., & Oswald, A. E. (2013). The effectiveness of team-based learning on learning outcomes in health professions education: BEME Guide No. 30. *Medical Teacher, 35*(12), e1608–1624. https://doi.org/10.3109/0142159x.2013.849802

Freeman, S., Eddy, S. L., McDonough, M., Smith, M. K., Okoroafor, N., Jordt, H., & Wenderoth, M. P. (2014). Active learning increases student performance in science, engineering, and mathematics. *Proceedings of the National Academy of Sciences of the United States of America, 111*(23), 8410–8415. https://doi.org/10.1073/pnas.1319030111

Goh, H. S., Zhang, H., Lee, C. N., Wu, X. V., & Wang, W. (2019). Value of nursing objective structured clinical examinations: A scoping review. *Nurse Educator, 44*(5), E1–E6. https://doi.org/10.1097/nne.0000000000000620

Gooblar, D. (2019, January 15). *Is it ever ok to lecture?* https://www.chronicle.com/article/is-it-ever-ok-to-lecture/

Hagler, D., & Morris, B. (2022). Learning environment and teaching methods. In M. H. Oermann, J. C. De Gagne, & B. C. Phillips (Eds.), *Teaching in nursing and role of the educator: The complete guide to best practice in teaching, evaluation, and curriculum development* (3rd ed., pp. 63–92). Springer Publishing Company.

Hong, S., & Yu, P. (2017). Comparison of the effectiveness of two styles of case-based learning implemented in lectures for developing nursing students' critical thinking ability: A randomized controlled trial. *International Journal of Nursing Studies, 68*, 16–24. https://doi.org/10.1016/j.ijnurstu.2016.12.008

Hu, R., Gao, H., Ye, Y., Ni, Z., Jiang, N., & Jiang, X. (2018). Effectiveness of flipped classrooms in Chinese baccalaureate nursing education: A meta-analysis of randomized controlled trials. *International Journal of Nursing Studies, 79*, 94–103. https://doi.org/10.1016/j.ijnurstu.2017.11.012

Kalaian, S. A., & Kasim, R. M. (2017). Effectiveness of various innovative learning methods in health science classrooms: A meta-analysis. *Advances in Health Sciences*

Education, 22(5), 1151–1167. https://doi .org/10.1007/s10459-017-9753-6

Koh, Y. Y. J., Schmidt, H. G., Low-Beer, N., & Rotgans, J. I. (2020). Team-based learning analytics: An empirical case study. *Academic Medicine, 95*(6), 872–878. https:// doi.org/10.1097/acm.0000000000003157

Li, S., Ye, X., & Chen, W. (2019). Practice and effectiveness of "nursing case-based learning" course on nursing student's critical thinking ability: A comparative study. *Nurse Education in Practice, 36*, 91–96. https://doi .org/10.1016/j.nepr.2019.03.007

Li, Y., Wang, X., Zhu, X. R., Zhu, Y. X., & Sun, J. (2019). Effectiveness of problem-based learning on the professional communication competencies of nursing students and nurses: A systematic review. *Nurse Education in Practice, 37*, 45–55. https://doi .org/10.1016/j.nepr.2019.04.015

Makhene, A. (2019). The use of the Socratic inquiry to facilitate critical thinking in nursing education. *Health SA Gesondheid, 24*, 1224. https://doi.org/10.4102/hsag.v24i0.1224

McLean, S. F. (2016). Case-based learning and its application in medical and health-care fields: A review of worldwide literature. *Journal of Medical Education and Curriculum Development, 3*, 39–49. https:// doi.org/10.4137/jmecd.S20377

Merisier, S., Larue, C., & Boyer, L. (2018). How does questioning influence nursing students' clinical reasoning in problem-based learning? A scoping review. *Nurse Education Today, 65*, 108–115. https://doi .org/10.1016/j.nedt.2018.03.006

Michaelsen, L. K., Parmelee, D. X., McMahon, K. K., & Levine, R. E. (2008). *Team based learning for health professions education: A guide to using small groups for improving learning.* Stylus.

Oermann, M. H. (2018). Wanted: Evidence to guide clinical teaching. *Nurse Educator, 43*(5), 223. https://doi.org/10.1097/ nne.0000000000000594

Oermann, M. H. (2020). Nursing education research: A new era. *Nurse Educator, 45*(3), 115. https://doi.org/10.1097/ nne.0000000000000830

Oermann, M. H. (2022). Evidence-based teaching in nursing. In M. H. Oermann, J. C. De Gagne, & B. C. Phillips (Eds.), *Teaching in nursing and role of the educator: The complete guide to best practice in teaching, evaluation, and curriculum development* (3rd ed., pp. 377–393). Springer Publishing Company.

Oermann, M. H., & Gaberson, K. (2021). *Evaluation and testing in nursing education* (6th ed.). Springer Publishing Company.

Oermann, M. H., Shellenbarger, T., & Gaberson, K. B. (2018). *Clinical teaching strategies in nursing* (5th ed.). Springer Publishing Company.

Phillips, N., & Duke, M. (2001). The questioning skills of clinical teachers and preceptors: A comparative study. *Journal of Advanced Nursing, 33*(4), 523–529. https://doi .org/10.1046/j.1365-2648.2001.01682.x

Phillips, N. M., Duke, M. M., & Weerasuriya, R. (2017). Questioning skills of clinical facilitators supporting undergraduate nursing students. *Journal of Clinical Nursing, 26*(23-24), 4344–4352. https://doi .org/10.1111/jocn.13761

Profetto-McGrath, J., Bulmer Smith, K., Day, R. A., & Yonge, O. (2004). The questioning skills of tutors and students in a context based baccalaureate nursing program. *Nurse Education Today, 24*(5), 363–372. https://doi.org/https://doi.org/10.1016/j .nedt.2004.03.004

Reimschisel, T., Herring, A. L., Huang, J., & Minor, T. J. (2017). A systematic review of the published literature on team-based learning in health professions education. *Medical Teacher, 39*(12), 1227–1237. https://doi.org/10.1080/01421 59x.2017.1340636

Sayyah, M., Shirbandi, K., Saki-Malehi, A., & Rahim, F. (2017). Use of a problem-based learning teaching model for undergraduate medical and nursing education: A systematic review and meta-analysis. *Advances in Medical Education and Practice, 8*, 691–700. https://doi.org/10.2147/amep .S143694

Selim, A. A., & Dawood, E. (2015). Objective structured video examination in psychiatric and mental health nursing: A learning and assessment method. *Journal of Nursing Education, 54*(2), 87–95. https://doi.org/10.3928/01484834-20150120-04

Sisk, R. J. (2011). Team-based learning: Systematic research review. *Journal of Nursing Education, 50*(12), 665–669. https://doi.org/10.3928/01484834-20111017-01

Theobald, E. J., Hill, M. J., Tran, E., Agrawal, S., Arroyo, E. N., Behling, S., Chambwe, N., Cintrón, D. L., Cooper, J. D., Dunster, G., Grummer, J. A., Hennessey, K., Hsiao, J., Iranon, N., Jones, L., 2nd, Jordt, H., Keller, M., Lacey, M. E., Littlefield, C. E., Lowe, A., Newman, S., Okolo, V., Olroyd, S., Peecook, B. R., Pickett, S. B., Slager, D. L., Caviedes-Solis, I. W., Stanchak, K. E., Sundaravardan, V., Valdebenito, C., Williams, C. R., Zinsli, K., & Freeman, S. (2020). Active learning narrows achievement gaps for underrepresented students in undergraduate science, technology, engineering, and math. *Proceedings of the National Academy of Sciences of the United States of America, 117*(12), 6476–6483. https://doi.org/10.1073/pnas.1916903117

Thistlethwaite, J. E., Davies, D., Ekeocha, S., Kidd, J. M., MacDougall, C., Matthews, P., Purkis, J., & Clay, D. (2012). The effectiveness of case-based learning in health professional education. A BEME systematic review: *BEME Guide* No. 23. *Medical Teacher, 34*(6), e421–444. https://doi.org/10.3109/0142159x.2012.680939

Vacek, J., & Liesveld, J. (2020). Teaching concepts to nursing students using model case studies, the Venn diagram, and questioning strategies. *Nursing Education Perspectives, 41*(6), 373–375. https://doi.org/10.1097/01.NEP.0000000000000514

Ward, M., Knowlton, M. C., & Laney, C. W. (2018). The flip side of traditional nursing education: A literature review. *Nurse Education in Practice, 29*, 163–171. https://doi.org/10.1016/j.nepr.2018.01.003

Wosinski, J., Belcher, A. E., Dürrenberger, Y., Allin, A.-C., Stormacq, C., & Gerson, L. (2018). Facilitating problem-based learning among undergraduate nursing students: A qualitative systematic review. *Nurse Education Today, 60*, 67–74. https://doi.org/https://doi.org/10.1016/j.nedt.2017.08.015

Xu, P., Chen, Y., Nie, W., Wang, Y., Song, T., Li, H., Li, J., Yi, J., & Zhao, L. (2019). The effectiveness of a flipped classroom on the development of Chinese nursing students' skill competence: A systematic review and meta-analysis. *Nurse Education Today, 80*, 67–77. https://doi.org/10.1016/j.nedt.2019.06.005

8

Resources to Support Program Goal Attainment: Essential to Achieve Excellence and Distinction in Nursing Education

Marsha Howell Adams, PhD, RN, CNE, FAAN, ANEF

Karen Frith, PhD, RN, NEC-BC, CNE

Amelia S. Lanz, EdD, RN, CNE

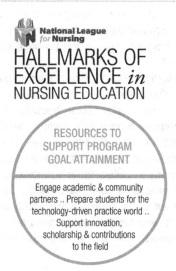

National League for Nursing

HALLMARKS OF EXCELLENCE *in* NURSING EDUCATION

RESOURCES TO SUPPORT PROGRAM GOAL ATTAINMENT

Engage academic & community partners .. Prepare students for the technology-driven practice world .. Support innovation, scholarship & contributions to the field

INTRODUCTION

Having adequate physical, human, and financial resources – and using them effectively – is essential for a school or program to achieve excellence and distinction. Resource management includes managing current resources as well as developing strategies to obtain new resources to support the goals of the strategic plan (Giddens & Morton,

2018). This chapter addresses resources to support program goal attainment and focuses on the importance of partnerships, technology, student support services, ongoing faculty development, and fiscal resources as essential to achieve excellence and become a nursing program of distinction. Resources are essential to support faculty as they develop innovative, evidence-based strategies to facilitate teaching and learning and to engage students in the learning process (see Chapters 3 and 7). They also are key to supporting scholarly efforts (see Chapter 9), designing and implementing innovative curricula (see Chapter 6), enhancing the ongoing development of faculty and staff (see Chapter 4), supporting effective institutional and professional leadership (see Chapter 10), and facilitating continuous quality improvement (see Chapter 5).

ACADEMIC PRACTICE PARTNERSHIPS: A VALUABLE RESOURCE FOR PROMOTING EXCELLENCE AND DISTINCTION

Strong academic practice partnerships are essential for promoting excellence and moving nursing education programs forward in their quest for distinction, and they are developed and strengthened through the allocation of resources. Academic practice partnerships are collaborative relationships between nursing education programs and practice settings that are based on a continuing commitment, mutual respect, a shared vision and goals, strong communication, and collective knowledge (Beal et al., 2012). They are "mechanism[s] for advancing nursing practice to improve the health of the public" (Beal et al., 2012, p. 328).

In 2011, the Institute of Medicine (IOM) of the National Academy of Sciences released *The Future of Nursing: Leading Change, Advancing Health*. In this groundbreaking report, the nursing profession was challenged to become "full partners with physicians and other health professionals in redesigning health care in the United States" (p. 7). Nursing education programs, in addition to healthcare organizations and others, were tasked with providing opportunities to promote the development of nurse leaders and academic practice partnerships to collaboratively participate in this healthcare transformation. Nursing education programs have the potential to contribute to this transformation in incredibly significant ways, particularly in the areas of patient-centered care, research, clinical innovation, and leadership. Nursing administrators and faculty may consider the following Indicators when addressing this Hallmark of Excellence in Nursing Education©:

▹ What are the criteria used to determine the agencies/organizations with which the nursing program will partner?

▹ How are partners engaged with faculty members and students to achieve excellence in the nursing program?

Developing and sustaining academic practice partnerships has been a strong focus of the National League for Nursing (NLN) and the American Association of Colleges of Nursing (AACN). In 2013, the NLN introduced the Accelerating to Practice initiative. The purpose of this initiative was to create partnerships among not-for-profit organizations and private enterprise to develop innovative programs that better prepared nursing students as they transitioned into practice (Tagliareni, 2013). A group of prominent nurse educators and hospital administrators who had existing academic practice partnerships came together to develop new curriculum models that address readiness for practice, innovative orientation programs using simulation, and faculty strategies to create collaborative learning experiences.

In 2012, AACN partnered with the American Organization of Nurse Leaders (AONL) (formerly the American Organization of Nurse Executives [AONE]) to develop guiding principles related to creating academic practice partnerships. These principles can assist a nursing education program in recognizing what agencies/organizations are the best fit to develop a dynamic partnership. These guiding principles emphasize collaboration, respect and trust, knowledge, commitment for nurses to work within their fullest scope of practice, commitment to nurses for a smooth transition from education to practice, commitment for processes to recognize life-long learning, and creation of a database for collecting and analyzing nursing workforce data (AACN & AONE, 2012).

When a nursing education program is in the early stages of engaging in a possible academic practice partnership, consideration should be given to the extent to which the following factors exist:

- Mutual knowledge regarding the college/school of nursing and the partnering organization and what each entity can bring to the table including resources
- The initiatives the college/school of nursing and the partnering organization might pursue that would be of greatest benefit to both
- Shared vision
- Identification of necessary key players
- Development of a business case which includes addressing the cost and return on investment for each of the institutions involved and whether this investment is mutually valued financially

In subsequent interactions, other items need to be considered such as clear goals, timeline and outcomes for the initiative, consultation from external experts that might be needed, and consideration of the environment regarding time, space, regulation, and funding. AACN and AONE (2012) have developed a template to use when developing partnership initiatives.

In 2016, AACN published *Advancing Healthcare Transformation: A New Era for Academic Nursing*, which examined the potential for possible partnerships between colleges/schools of nursing and academic health centers (AHCs). One of the report findings was that "insufficient resources are a barrier to supporting a significantly enhanced role for academic nursing" (AACN, 2016, p. 2). An example of an insufficient resource is tuition and college fee-dependent funding structures. The funding structure for colleges/schools of nursing at times limits the ability to participate in academic practice partnerships due to lack of funding to support nursing education and practice initiatives.

A number of exemplar colleges/schools of nursing and healthcare organizations are highlighted in this document (AACN, 2016). It must be noted that this work focused on academic practice partnerships between colleges/schools of nursing and AHCs, but these principles are applicable to colleges/schools of nursing that are not affiliated with AHCs . . . and to practice settings such as home care agencies, community centers, public schools, and other settings where nursing practice occurs that are not AHCs.

Implementation of successful academic practice partnerships can better prepare nursing students for practice, advance nursing practice, improve the quality of patient care provided, and improve health outcomes. The engagement between partners, faculty, and students can help to accomplish strategic goals moving nursing programs closer to achieving excellence and distinction.

The literature provides numerous examples of successful academic practice partnerships between colleges/schools of nursing and healthcare organizations. In 2012, Beal published an integrative review on academic practice partnerships which included 110 articles focusing on key elements needed for successful partnerships, partnership benefits, faculty practice, types of partnerships including improvement of care to diverse populations, quality education to students and agency staff, development of potential research trajectories, transformation of nursing education, and nursing workforce issues. While most of these articles were anecdotal, they documented successful results and benefits of forming such collaborations and illustrated how visionary thinking can lead to exciting outcomes.

MacPhee (2009) developed an academic practice partnership logic model including inputs, activities, outputs, and outcomes needed to have a successful partnership. The items identified supported those areas identified by the AACN and AONE task force described earlier in the chapter including a common philosophy and vision, identifying short- and long-term goals, and identifying individuals who will champion the cause for academic practice partnerships. In this logic model, dedicated time and resources, both human and fiscal, were found to be especially important to accomplish identified activities and projects. The partnership described by this author created educational workshops, academic appointments for practicing nurses, transition plans for nurses moving from education to the practice setting, and research nursing collaborations.

Howard et al. (2020) describes an academic practice partnership where a teaching model is implemented using a logic model with the common goal being to increase the number of doctorally prepared advanced practice nurses (APN). The teaching model involved appointing doctorally prepared nurses from the practice setting as adjunct faculty and pairing them with nursing faculty teaching in the Doctor of Nursing Practice (DNP) courses. This strategy was found to enhance student learning outcomes and provide some relief for the nursing faculty shortage. Resources identified as crucial included financial, faculty, staff, classrooms, technology, simulation, clinical sites, and materials for faculty preparation related to the teaching model (p. 287). It was reported that both students and faculty were very satisfied with the model outcomes.

In an effort to provide a smooth transition from the student role to practicing registered nurse, Trepanier et al. (2017) describes an academic practice partnership between a college of nursing and a healthcare organization that designed and implemented a nurse residency program. In this partnership, all students from that college with plans to work in the hospital where the partnership existed participated in the residency program, which began during the students' last semester capstone course. The academic and practice representatives worked together to design the capstone course, which included identifying 29 competencies that were needed to be met during the capstone course. The results were that all who participated were able to meet the competencies. Positive outcomes were achieved including better prepared registered nurses as measured by a series of assessments, metrics, and evaluations; a decrease in the practice organization's turnover rate, which led to cost savings for the health organization; and development of a set of competencies that will better prepare nursing students for transition into practice.

TECHNOLOGY TO FACILITATE, SUPPORT, AND EVALUATE STUDENT LEARNING

Nursing faculty who strive for excellence use educational and healthcare technologies to prepare students with information literacy, informatics skills, and clinical skills/competencies to thrive in practice. This Hallmark calls for visionary leadership and innovative faculty to normalize risk-taking using educational technology. The first decision about technology is the most important: Programs need to invest in highly usable technology resources, which means selecting technology that promotes the achievement of student learning outcomes effectively, efficiently, and satisfactorily. Coupled with faculty who routinely try new teaching approaches using technology, student learning and engagement flourishes (Njie-Carr et al., 2017). In addition, a curriculum with planned informatics content and competencies assessments gives students the best opportunity to become practice-ready nurses (Harerimana & Mtshali, 2020).

Nursing faculty who wish to achieve this Hallmark might ask themselves:

> How are faculty members and students prepared for/supported in the use of technology to facilitate and evaluate learning?

> What commitment has the nursing program made to integrate the use of technology throughout the program?

> To what extent is informatics integrated throughout the program to ensure that students are prepared for the current technology-driven practice world?

Technology to Support Learning

Research on educational technology has shown that students from all disciplines learn as well or better in technology-enhanced environments than traditional classroom delivery (Brown Wilson et al., 2020). In nursing, results from a national mixed methods study on quality Indicators in nursing education showed "programs incorporating hybrid learning strategies were significantly more likely to have higher NCLEX pass rates" than traditional or online-only programs (Spector et al., 2020, p. S30). So, what does this finding mean for nursing schools/programs? It suggests that the Hallmark related to the integration of planned and well-executed educational technology in the classroom and beyond is critical to achieving excellence in nursing education.

Faculty support for educational technologies must be in place for technology to facilitate learning rather than stymie it. Resources include "smart" classroom equipment, video recording devices, software and support, equipment for high- and low-fidelity laboratory experiences, supplies for laboratory equipment, and maintenance agreements for equipment. Those resources can be categorized into technology-enhanced teaching approaches: flipped classrooms, online courses, and simulation. Implementing flipped classrooms and online courses requires faculty time to develop content, produce audio/video recordings, and create meaningful assessments before class; however, lack of technology support for these innovative approaches is often reported in research findings (Njie-Carr et al., 2017). When educational technology is used in flipped classrooms, students are engaged in class activities, have better learning outcomes, and express better satisfaction with the course (Njie-Carr et al., 2017). However, nursing faculty need to be mindful of the work assigned when designing online courses or flipped classrooms. Northrup-Snyder et al. (2020) found online nursing courses required on average 6 to 24 more hours per week than the Department of Education recommendations for 3-credit hour courses.

Simulation in nursing education should be based on standards published by the International Nursing Association for Clinical Simulation and Learning (INACSL Standards Committee, 2017) that require systems such as providing personnel to support the simulation program; using a system to manage space and equipment; and maintaining the financial resources to support stability, sustainability, and growth of the simulation program. Years of careful planning to implement and evaluate simulation in nursing education may be needed to incorporate the best practices. Programs of distinction take additional steps to become certified (Society for Simulation in Healthcare, 2021) or accredited (Society for Simulation in Healthcare, 2020).

Research on simulation is plentiful. Early efforts focused on student satisfaction, but as INACSL simulation standards developed and the National Council of State Boards of Nursing (NCSBB) recognized simulation as a partial replacement for clinical experiences (Hayden et al., 2014), many quasi-experimental and experimental studies were conducted to access other outcomes. Among the outcomes assessed were confidence, which was shown to improve (Moxley et al., 2021; Turrise et al., 2020); clinical proficiency, which was enhanced (Hardenberg et al., 2020; Scalon da Costa et al., 2019); clinical practice, which was safer (Craig et al., 2021; Turner, 2020); and perceived value of interprofessional practice, which was found to increase (Marion-Martins & Pinho, 2020).

Commitment to Integrate Technology in Program

Program administrators must allocate resources to support the integration of technology to enhance students' learning experiences. Spector et al. (2020) found at-risk nursing programs often lacked resources to facilitate nursing education including information technology, simulation, and laboratory supplies. Time for faculty development and experimentation with educational technology is also a necessary consideration (Roney et al., 2017). In addition, technology support for students and availability of high-speed Internet access at home must be considered as essential components to a technology-enhanced nursing curriculum (Frith, 2020a).

Teaching telehealth and mobile health applications became a necessary strategy during the COVID-19 pandemic. Authors reported on the use of various virtual clinical experiences for undergraduate and graduate students, which show promise for continued use after students' return to clinical settings (Chike-Harris et al., 2020; DeFoor et al., 2020; Fogg et al., 2020; Foronda et al., 2020; Posey et al., 2020; Powers et al., 2020; Robinson-Reilly et al., 2020; Walsh, 2020). Each of the experiences with informatics content and learning activities prepare students to be safe and competent nurses for healthcare settings saturated with technology.

Program administrators and faculty need to consider the usability of technology (U.S. Department of Health & Human Services, 2020) before any purchase is made. IT experts also need to serve as consultants to assist in vendor selection and technical implementation of the system or software. This attention to the selection, purchase, and implementation of educational technology is critical because a bad purchase decision will cost a sizeable amount of money and leave faculty and students frustrated (Koivisto et al., 2018). Koivisto and colleagues developed a game that simulated practice and required nursing students to develop clinical reasoning skills; the game was based on the following design principles: (1) integrate learning outcomes with the game mechanics; (2) create authentic patient scenarios; (3) use graphics, animations, audio, and video; (4) create opportunities for interactions in realistic settings; (5) provide options that allow for experimentation; and (6) embed reflection-in-action by providing feedback. While most nursing faculty may not develop their own games, the design principles can be used to evaluate which educational games and simulations to use in the teaching/learning process.

Informatics in Nursing Programs

The Essentials: Core Competencies for Professional Nursing Education (AACN, 2021) identifies Information Management and Healthcare Technologies as an essential domain in nursing education. The domain is defined as "information and communication technologies and informatics processes used to provide care, gather data, form information to drive decision making, and support professionals as they expand knowledge and wisdom for practice. Informatics processes and technologies are used to manage and improve the delivery of safe, high-quality, and efficient healthcare services in accordance with best practice and professional and regulatory standards" (AACN, 2020, p. 12). The fact that Information Management and Healthcare Technologies is one of the 10 *Essentials* demonstrates the importance of integrating these concepts through all baccalaureate nursing curricula.

Even though standards for nursing education call for nurses to be competent using informatics knowledge and skills, integrating informatics courses and content is not ubiquitous. Bove (2020) replicated a study re-examining the integration of informatics in nursing curricula from the top 25 nursing programs from the *U.S. News and World Report*. As compared to the initial findings reported by Hunter et al. (2013) seven years earlier, Bove found an increase of informatics content integration in master's and doctoral programs, but not in baccalaureate programs. Studies on the barriers to and facilitators of integrating informatics into nursing curricula have consistent findings: (1) Faculty need time to learn informatics concepts, (2) faculty need peers or a champion with informatics expertise to support integration of these concepts into curricula, (3) faculty need technology support, and (4) faculty need educational technology tools appropriate for teaching students to be practice ready (Forman et al., 2020; Foster & Sethares, 2017; Fulton et al., 2014).

The informatics concepts needed in nursing curricula have changed over the past two decades beginning with teaching computer skills and focusing on teaching information management skills for electronic health records with the passage of *the Health Information Technology for Economic and Clinical Health Act (HITECH)* in 2009 (Skiba, 2017). However, today's students also need informatics skills for connected care which include mobile health applications, telehealth, health monitoring using body and environmental sensors, and home-based healthcare technologies that connect providers and patients (Frith, 2019a, 2019b, 2020b, 2021a, 2021b). To teach students how to use these health information technologies, faculty need access to the same technologies used in healthcare settings in their nursing laboratories.

STUDENT SUPPORT SERVICES ARE CULTURALLY SENSITIVE AND EMPOWER STUDENTS

Student support services typically encompass a variety of resources focused on meeting students' needs and fostering their success. These programs may be housed within the nursing school/college itself and/or within the larger institutional setting. Such support services include those related to recruitment, retention, progression, graduation, and career planning. Because students come to the academic setting with diverse backgrounds — social, economic, developmental, educational, and experiential — an innovative, comprehensive approach is needed to meet this Hallmark and achieve excellence in the school/program. Program development that will meet the needs of a diverse student population call on faculty and administrators to consider the following Hallmark Indicators:

> To what extent do students report that the recruitment and admission process was a welcoming one that acknowledged their unique needs?

> To what extent do students express comfort about seeking out and using the student services that are available to them?

> To what extent do students report satisfaction with the extent of support they receive throughout the program, at graduation, and in relation to entering a new career?

The organization of student support services varies by institution. Common expectations and responsibilities include assisting students in the successful transition to college, assisting in the procurement of adequate financial resources, and providing programs and services for students who experience academic challenges or disabilities. Also, student support services often focus on helping individuals thrive outside of classrooms through initiatives such as leadership skill development, diversity awareness, recreation and campus community life, career planning, service learning, and student health. A primary goal is to support student success through a seamless educational experience (National Association of Student Personnel Administrators, Inc., 1987).

It is important that the nursing school/college collaborate with various support units across the institution to develop resources and quality programs that support individuals and groups of students. The Council for the Advancement of Standards in Higher Education (CAS, 2019) indicates that a holistic student learning experience is best achieved when student support professionals team with faculty/academic affairs to develop programs and assessments. According to O'Halloran (2019), "The current movement in education to bring learning beyond the strictly cognitive process to one that is dynamic and social is at the heart of collaboration, as both speak to meeting the needs of the whole student" (p. 307). Collaborative efforts have been recognized as having a positive impact on student retention and persistence (Syno et al., 2019). In addition, collaborative efforts can help ensure that resources and services are integrated to facilitate student navigation (O'Halloran, 2019).

The effectiveness of support programs, including departmental performance Indicators and student attitudes and feelings related to the quality of services, should be consistently evaluated (Schuh et al., 2016; Ursinus College, 2015). Quantitative measures can include items such as acceptance rates, retention rates, number of scheduled campus visits, number of financial aid applications processed, number of students accessing support services, and student exit data. Qualitative measures may include perceived satisfaction with various services and processes, helpfulness and support of admissions staff, the usefulness of counseling and advising services, student satisfaction with technical support, and surveys of program satisfaction. To determine the focus for development and planning, needs assessments can also be incorporated (Schuh et al., 2016; Ursinus College, 2015). The preceding are merely illustrative examples rather than an exhaustive list as the possibilities are extensive. The Hallmark Indicators previously described can easily be targeted through the assessment process.

Admission services at both the institution and program level should function with clear goals that reflect the institutional/program mission (CAS, 2019). Processes relevant to admission and enrollment should be clearly articulated for potential students and address their unique needs (first time undergraduate, transfer, testing-entrance exam options, financial support). Institution and program information regarding admission policies, application and decision timelines, and support resources must be current and accurate (CAS, 2019). Resources may include information pertaining to testing services, entrance exam preparation, credential/certification assistance, program policies, and opportunities beyond the classroom (i.e., support groups, clubs, organizations).

College admission criteria has become an area of focused scrutiny over the last several years. Traditional college entrance exams (ACT, SAT) have been questioned as a valid predictor of college success, especially for disadvantaged and minority students (Furuta, 2017). A more holistic approach to the admissions process has been a point of appeal. For nursing education, evidence suggests that standardized program preadmission exam scores (e.g., HESI A2 & ATI Test of Essential Academic Skills [TEAS]) and preadmission GPA do correlate with a higher likelihood of success (Elkins, 2015; Zamanzadeh et al., 2020). Others have recognized that personal characteristics, including values and interests, should be considered in the selection process, arguing that academic capability alone is insufficient for the nursing role (Pitt et al., 2014). Graduate education is not without exception as admission tests like the Graduate Record Exam (GRE) have been associated with poor predictability and identified as a barrier to student enrollment (Katz et al., 2009). Determining admission criteria that correlates with student success is an area in need of innovation and requires investigation according to nurse researchers (Capponi & Barber, 2020).

In whatever way the admission process is organized, in today's educational environment, the need for diversity among nursing student enrollment has been well established. Diversity embraces differences in age; sex; race; ethnicity; sexual orientation; gender identity; family structures; geographic locations; national origin; immigrants and refugees; language; physical, functional, and learning abilities; religious beliefs; and socioeconomic status (AACN, 2017). Optimal nursing care hinges on a workforce that reflects the expanding diversity of the population. The important benefits for nursing and health care include enhanced cultural competence, better access for minority patients and underserved communities, and expanded minority research initiatives (LaVeist & Pierre, 2014; Phillips & Malone, 2014). Therefore, support services should be comprehensively developed to assist diverse students as well as those who do not encompass minorities. It is important to note that inclusive institutions strive to have a faculty, staff, and administration that reflects diversity. According to the U.S. Department of Education (U.S. DOE, 2016), students need to see themselves reflected in the faculty and the curriculum to promote a sense of belonging and inclusion. Institutions should implement strategies to increase their leadership, faculty, staff, and students' cultural competency to create an all-encompassing college environment with effective support services (U.S. DOE, 2016).

Recruitment may be implemented using a variety of strategies. Outreach programs at elementary and secondary school levels within the local community is one example. Murray et al. (2016) implemented a successful high school career academy focused on preparing students from minority settings for nursing program admission. The program also included strategies for student retention after admission to nursing school. Advising and peer support programs to help students negotiate key areas such as financial application submissions and standardized exam preparation have been deemed helpful (Murray et al., 2016). Cost is often a barrier to higher education. Comprehensive programs to assist students with financial resources, including federal aid programs, scholarship programs, grant funding, loan repayment programs, and disadvantaged student funds, can help eliminate barriers (U.S. DOE, 2016).

Unfortunately, nursing education is associated with high rates of attrition on a global scale (Mooring, 2016). A multidimensional approach to support retention and persistence is needed for all students – pre-licensure, post-RN, and graduate – and for students enrolled via different formats – in-person, online/virtual/distance, full-time, part-time, and so on. Strategies that include opportunities for socialization and personal support (coaching, life management skills) have resulted in positive outcomes for diverse students (Mooring, 2016). Both peer and faculty mentoring programs have been shown to support academic success, improve engagement, and promote a sense of connectedness (Balzer Carr & London, 2019). Additional strategies could include support from a retention specialist, comprehensive orientation programs, and remedial assistance (Bumby, 2020). Identifying at-risk students early and developing a support plan is recommended for all forms of program (Balzer Carr & London, 2019; Gazza & Hunker, 2014). Distance programs should include targeted retention strategies that focus on advising, technological skill readiness, ongoing assessment to enhance course and program delivery, and comprehensive orientations (Gazza & Hunker, 2014). Practical strategies developed by student affairs personnel at one institution to assist online learners included the use of course management systems to track student engagement, regular communication with students to assess progress, individualized coaching, and the availability of support services outside the standard 8 to 5 hours . . . all of which could be applied to the traditional setting (Doyle, 2020). The author also noted that participation in orientation and regular class attendance were important factors that positively influence retention.

Student support services need to be configured to meet various needs for a diverse mixture of students. These services should work in tandem with the educational curriculum to prepare students for the workplace. Career service programs that extend beyond resume writing and job fair offerings to support skill development in leadership, teamwork, communication, professionalism, and critical thinking can arm students with the tools to succeed (Arnold, 2018). Providing opportunities for student growth and development in these areas over the educational course is necessary. Career services should help build connections and partnerships to engage students and stakeholders (Arnold, 2018). In nursing, additional elements should be considered as entry into the workplace is associated with significant challenges. Transition-to-practice (TTP) programs and nurse residency programs are recommended to ease novice nurse transition (NCSBB, 2014). Career guidance in nursing programs can connect students with TTP opportunities. Collaboration with practice partners can be undertaken to expand these opportunities for students. APNs must be prepared to face challenges in the workplace readily. According to Kopf et al. (2018), competency-based transition programs are also effective for the APN career transition.

Support services and resources must be innovative and well-planned to help students effectively manage the challenges of the educational environment. The necessity for a holistic approach that appreciates the diverse needs of individuals is well-established in the literature. Regular assessments should be conducted to determine the extent to which these goals are achieved.

FINANCIAL RESOURCES TO SUPPORT COLLEGE/SCHOOL INITIATIVES

In addition to the resources already described – academic-clinical partnerships, technology, and student support services – financial resources to support other activities and initiatives needed for program goal attainment also are essential to position the nursing school/program to achieve excellence and distinction. While the management of financial resources in a college/school of nursing is a key responsibility of the dean/director and their administrative team, faculty and staff also need to be cognizant of the resources that are available, how they are allocated and can be used, and how to request funding for new projects/initiatives. All members of the academic community need to understand how major stakeholders (e.g., the parent institution and communities of interest) value and are invested in the college/school's mission, vision, goals, and core values, as well as understand the following:

> To what extent do financial resources support
>> visionary, long-range planning and creative initiatives?
>> faculty development and certification as a nurse educator?
>> continuous quality improvement of the program?

- To what extent do resources available to faculty members, students, and administrators support efforts to be innovative, continually develop as members of the nursing profession and the academic community, and enact needed change?
- In what ways does the institution provide resources to support faculty scholarly endeavors such as grant writing, publications, and presentations at regional and national conferences?
- What administrative and financial support is available for faculty members to be innovative and evidence based in their approach to teaching and learning as well as in their approach to the design, implementation, and evaluation of the curriculum?
- How do faculty members' workloads support their efforts to create a preferred future for nursing education, nursing practice, or nursing research?

Students, faculty, staff, and administrators are all affected by the number of financial resources available to support college/school initiatives. Financial resources are needed to secure productive faculty, both tenure and clinical track, who can be successful in the roles of teaching, research/scholarship, service, and/or practice. These resources are needed to promote faculty development as teachers, scholars, practitioners, and research scientists. A diverse student body requires additional resources focusing on recruitment and retention strategies and student initiatives that will promote the development of future professional nurses, APNs, and doctorally prepared nurses.

For a college/school of nursing to experience productive growth and development, a nursing program wants "to predict the needs of a school beyond the next one to two years, and make transparent, value-based decisions" (Broome et al., 2018, p. 97). Giddens and Morton (2018) recommended developing partnerships with deans and directors of other colleges/schools to develop initiatives where resources could be shared. Universities are now collaborating with community colleges to create dual nursing programs where students can obtain their associate degree and baccalaureate degree simultaneously. Other universities are collaborating in the development of joint programs such as a joint nursing science PhD program where financial resources can be shared.

Broome et al. (2018) describe a business development initiative (BDI) to support education, research, and professional development of faculty. The BDI served as a method of relying on non-tuition revenue from workshops and course offerings outside the realm of the program of study, as a resource to support programmatic needs, as well as faculty and staff development. This successful entrepreneurial initiative focused on the following crucial elements: mission related, margin focused, incentive alignment for faculty and staff, infrastructure, and return on investment (p. 99). While this initiative took place in a private university, it can be implemented effectively in public universities.

The financial resource Hallmark focuses on enhancing student success, faculty competence, innovation, and scholarly endeavors. Each of these areas has Indicators that nursing educators are encouraged to "think about" as they strive for excellence and pursue distinction.

It is imperative that financial resources (for faculty development with a focus on mentorship) be available to promote student success initiatives. In a review of research on successful student achievement (PR Group, 2014), 10 strategies were identified where faculty can support student success:

> Inquire about students' educational and professional career goals.

> Incorporate student goals into course assignments.

> Provide feedback about student performance on a regular basis.

> Clarify with students their understanding of course materials and direct them to available resources.

> Know your students' names.

> Ask for student feedback throughout the semester.

> Act as a professional role model.

> Provide opportunities for student relationships to develop where they can connect and support each other.

> Provide opportunities for students to share information about their backgrounds and cultural experiences.

> Provide opportunities for peer-to-peer support.

An example of how resources can successfully support student success is seen at the University of Alabama in Huntsville where the College of Nursing was able to create a retention and persistence program for underrepresented and at-risk students using a three-prong approach which included the use of a synthetic human simulator that students interact with during anatomy and physiology courses to connect the dots between didactic content and actual interactive body systems, development of the English for Academic and Professional Purposes (EAPP) (https://www.uah.edu/nursing/about/eapp), and UR-STAR (Strategies, Training, and Resources) (https://www.uah.edu/nursing/students/student-organizations/ur-star) initiatives. The EAPP initiative focuses on intensive language and culture strategies with faculty coaches, while UR-STAR provides faculty support and faculty/student and peer-to-peer mentoring. This retention and persistence program is supported through grant funding from the Caring Foundation of Blue Cross Blue Shield of Alabama.

The NLN has identified nurse educator core competencies that nursing faculty can use to guide their growth and development as truly competent nursing faculty members. These competencies can be used to create annual faculty goals in relation to facilitating learning and learner development, assessment and evaluation strategies, innovative curriculum design, programmatic outcomes, continuous quality improvement, and leadership (Christensen & Simmons, 2020). Peer and senior faculty members can mentor novice faculty using these competencies as a basis for their mentorship. Resources can be used to develop centers for education and leadership excellence. An example is Duke University's School of Nursing Institute for Educational Excellence (https://nursing.duke.edu/centers-and-institutes/iee-institute-educational-excellence#) where preparing master teachers and developing nurse leaders and scholars to advance the science of nursing education takes place.

Nursing faculty can further validate these competencies by seeking certification as a nurse educator and applying as a fellow in the NLN Academy of Nursing Education. Resources are needed to support faculty in these endeavors. For example, if faculty have designated travel funds, could those travel funds be used to support the certification and/or fellowship costs? Chapter 11 provides more detail regarding opportunities to seek certification and fellowships.

The mission of the university and community college will determine the expectations for faculty scholarship. Some institutions have a stronger emphasis on teaching, while others focus more on research. Creating a culture of scholarship in your organization starts with the expectation that faculty will engage in scholarship. Resources are needed to support faculty scholarship. For example, administrators need to consider the strategic goals of the organization when hiring faculty. This will drive the hiring process as to what types of faculty are needed such as an established researcher with grant funding, a master teacher whose focus is nursing education research, an APN with a recognized practice, or a novice nurse faculty who shows potential for excelling in research/scholarship. Building a strong research initiative requires the hiring of productive research faculty and providing start-up funds, travel funds, staff such as a biostatistician, grant writing support, adequate release time, and other resources to support research such as hiring an associate dean of research, creating an office of research support, or developing a research center (Mundt, 2018). Supporting novice faculty with start-up funds can position those faculty in the development of a strong research trajectory (McBride et al., 2017).

CONCLUSION

Continually striving for excellence with the goal of attaining distinction should be on the forefront of all administrators, faculty, staff, and students. Excellence is a practice, a habit that is ingrained into every choice and action; as such, building a culture of excellence can be quite challenging. One key characteristic that must be present during this journey is the availability of adequate resources to support all aspects of the college/school of nursing. The development of strong academic practice partnerships can help to bring resources into the college/school. Resources can enable faculty to embrace a rich collection of technologies to create active teaching approaches that are aligned with current best practices. Resources can sustain student support services, promote faculty development, and support faculty as they pursue research and scholarship endeavors, as well as service opportunities.

References

American Association of Colleges of Nursing. (2016). *Advancing healthcare transformation: A new era for academic nursing.* https://www.aacnnursing.org/portals/42/publications/aacn-new-era-report.pdf

American Association of Colleges of Nursing. (2017). *Diversity, inclusion, and equity in academic nursing.* https://www.aacnnursing.org/Diversity-Inclusion/Publications-on-Diversity/Position-Statement

American Association of Colleges of Nursing. (2020). *Re-envisioning the AACN essentials task force.* https://www.aacnnursing.org/About-AACN/AACN-Governance/Committees-and-Task-Forces/Essentials

American Association of Colleges of Nursing. (2021). *The essentials: Core competencies for professional nursing education.* https://www.aacnnursing.org/Education-Resources/AACN-Essentials

American Association of Colleges of Nursing & American Organization of Nurse Executives. (2012). *Guiding principles to academic-practice partnerships.* https://www.aacnnursing.org/Academic-Practice-Partnerships/The-Guiding-Principles

Arnold, W. W. (2018). Strengthening college support services to improve student transitioning to careers. *Journal of College Teaching & Learning, 15*(1), 5–26. https://eric-ed-gov.elib.uah.edu/contentdelivery/servlet/ERICServlet?accno=EJ1186161

Balzer Carr, B., & London, R. A. (2019). The role of learning support services in university students' educational outcomes. *Journal of College Student Retention: Research, Theory & Practice, 21*(1), 78–104. http://doi.org/elib.uah.edu/10.1177/1521025117690159

Beal, J. (2012). Academic-service partnerships in nursing: An integrative review. *Nursing Research and Practice,* 2012, 1–9. https://doi.org/10.1155/2012/501564

Beal, J., Alt-White, A., Erickson, J., Everett, L., Fleshner, I., Karshmer, J., Swider, S., & Gale, S. (2012). Academic practice partnerships: A national dialogue. *Journal of Professional Nursing, 28*(6), 327–332. https://doi.org/10.1016/j.profnurs.2012.09.001

Bove, L. A. (2020). Integration of informatics content in baccalaureate and graduate nursing education: An updated status report. *Nurse Educator, 45*(4), 206–209. https://doi.org/10.1097/NNE.0000000000000734

Broome, M., Bowersox, D., & Relf, M. (2018). A new funding model for nursing education through business development initiatives. *Journal of Professional Nursing, 34*(2), 97–102. https://doi.org/10.1016/j.profnurs.2017.10.003

Brown Wilson, C., Slade, C., Wong, W. Y. A., & Peacock, A. (2020). Health care students experience of using digital technology in patient care: A scoping review of the literature. *Nurse Education Today,* 95. https://doi.org/10.1016/j.nedt.2020.104580

Bumby, J. C. (2020). Evidence-based interventions for retention of nursing Students: A review of the literature. *Nurse Educator, 45*(6), 312–315. https://doi-org.elib.uah.edu/10.1097/NNE.0000000000000797

Capponi, N., & Mason Barber, L. A. (2020). Undergraduate nursing program admission criteria: A scoping review of the literature. *Nurse Education Today, 92,* N.PAG. https://doi-org.elib.uah.edu/10.1016/j.nedt.2020.104519

Chike-Harris, K. E., Harmon, E., & van Ravenstein, K. (2020). Graduate nursing telehealth education: Assessment of a one-day immersion approach. *Nursing Education Perspectives, 41*(5), E35–E36. https://doi.org/10.1097/01.NEP.0000000000000526

Christensen, L., & Simmons, L. (2020). *The scope of practice for academic nurse educators and academic clinical nurse educators* (3rd ed.). National League for Nursing. https://doi.org/10.1016/j.nedt.2018.01.027

Council for the Advancement of Standards in Higher Education (2019). *Undergraduate Admissions Programs and Services.* CAS professional standards for higher education (10th Ed.). Washington, DC: Author.

Craig, S. J., Kastello, J. C., Cieslowski, B. J., & Rovnyak, V. (2021). Simulation strategies to increase nursing student clinical competence in safe medication administration practices: A quasi-experimental study. *Nurse Education Today,* 96. https://doi.org/10.1016/j.nedt.2020.104605

DeFoor, M., Darby, W., & Pierce, V. (2020). "Get connected": Integrating telehealth triage in a prelicensure clinical simulation. *Journal of Nursing Education, 59*(9), 518–521. https://doi.org/10.3928/01484834-20200817-08

Doyle, J. (2020). Fostering student success outside of online classes. Inside Higher Ed. https://www.insidehighered.com/advice/2020/04/07/whats-role-student-affairs-and-academic-support-staff-when-most-students-arent

Elkins, N. (2015). Predictors of retention and passing the national council licensure examination for registered nurses. *Open Journal of Nursing, 5*(3), 218–225. https://doi.org/10.4236/ojn.2015.53026

Fogg, N., Wilson, C., Trinka, M., Campbell, R., Thomson, A., Merritt, L., Tietze, M., & Prior, M. (2020). Transitioning from direct care to virtual clinical experiences during the COVID-19 pandemic. *Journal of*

Professional Nursing, 36(6), 685–691. https://doi.org/10.1016/j.profnurs .2020.09.012

Forman, T. M., Armor, D. A., & Miller, A. S. (2020). A review of clinical informatics competencies in nursing to inform best practices in education and nurse faculty development. *Nursing Education Perspectives, 41*(1), E3–E7. https://doi .org/10.1097/01.NEP.0000000000000588

Foronda, C. L., Crenshaw, N., Briones, P. L., Snowden, K., Griffin, M. A., & Mitzova-Vladinov, G. (2020). Teaching and learning the skill of intubation using telehealth glasses. *Clinical Simulation in Nursing, 40*, 31–35. https://doi.org/10.1016/j .ecns.2019.12.005

Foster, M., & Sethares, K. (2017). Current strategies to implement informatics into the nursing curriculum: An integrative review. *Online Journal of Nursing Informatics* (OJNI), *21*(3). https://elib.uah .edu/login?url=https://www-proquest -com.elib.uah.edu/scholarly-journals/ current-strategies-implement-informatics -into/docview/1984791063/ se-2?accountid=14476

Frith, K. H. (2019a). Artificial intelligence: What does it mean for nursing? *Nursing Education Perspectives, 40*(4). 261. https://doi .org/10.1097/01.NEP.0000000000000543

Frith, K. H. (2019b). Home-based technologies for aging in place: Implications for nursing education. *Nursing Education Perspectives, 40*(3), 194–195. https://doi.org/10.1097/01 .NEP.0000000000000505

Frith, K. H. (2020a). Assessment of online education: Part 1. *Nursing Education Perspectives, 41*(5), 320–321. https://doi .org/10.1097/01.NEP.0000000000000727

Frith, K. H. (2020b). Mobile technologies in clinical trials. *Nursing Education Perspectives, 41*(3), 199–200. https://doi. org/10.1097/01.NEP.0000000000000665

Frith, K. H. (2021a). Telehealth delivery model in the mainstream. *Nursing Education Perspectives, 42*(1), 65. https://doi. org/10.1097/01.nep.0000000000000769

Frith, K. H. (2021b). The Star Trek tricorder is here: Handheld imaging technology.

Nursing Education Perspectives, 42(2), 130. https://doi.org/10.1097/01 .NEP.0000000000000789

Fulton, C. R., Meek, J. A., & Walker, P. H. (2014). Faculty and organizational characteristics associated with informatics/ health information technology adoption in DNP programs. *Journal of Professional Nursing: Official Journal of the American Association of Colleges of Nursing, 30*(4), 292–299. https://doi.org/10.1016/j .profnurs.2014.01.004

Furuta, J. (2017). Rationalization and student/ school personhood in U.S. college admissions: The rise of test-optional policies, 1987 to 2015. *Sociology of Education, 90*(3), 236–254. http://doi.org .elib.uah.edu/10.1177/0038040717713583

Gazza, E. A., & Hunker, D. F. (2014). Facilitating student retention in online graduate nursing education programs: A review of the literature. *Nurse Education Today, 34*(7), 1125–1129. https://doi.org/elib.uah .edu/10.1016/j.nedt.2014.01.010

Giddens, J., & Morton, P. (2018). Pearls of wisdom for chief academic nursing leaders. *Journal of Professional Nursing, 34*(2), 75–81. https://doi.org/10.1016/j .profnurs.2017.10.002

Hardenberg, J., Rana, I., & Tori, K. (2020). Evaluating impact of repeated exposure to high fidelity simulation: Skills acquisition and stress levels in postgraduate critical care nursing students. *Clinical Simulation in Nursing, 48*, 96–102. https://doi.org/10 .1016/j.ecns.2020.06.002

Harerimana, A., & Mtshali, N. G. (2020). Using exploratory and confirmatory factor analysis to understand the role of technology in nursing education. *Nurse Education Today, 92*. https:// doi.org/10.1016/j.nedt.2020.104490.

Hayden, J. K., Smiley, R. A., Alexander, M., Kardong-Edgren, S., & Jeffries, P. R. (2014). The NCSBN National Simulation Study: A longitudinal, randomized, controlled study replacing clinical hours with simulation in prelicensure nursing education. *Journal of Nursing Regulation, 5*(2, Supplement), S3–S40. https://doi.org/10.1016/ S2155-8256(15)30062-4

Howard, P., Williams, T., El-Mallakh, P., Melander, S., Tharp-Barrie, K., Lock, S., & MacCallum, T. (2020). An innovative teaching model in an academic-practice partnership for a Doctor of Nursing Practice program. *Journal of Professional Nursing, 36*(5), 285–291. https://doi.org/10.1016/j .profnurs.2020.04.010

Hunter, K., McGonigle, D., & Hebda, T. (2013). The integration of informatics content in baccalaureate and graduate nursing education. *Nurse Educator, 38*(3), 110–116. https://doi.org/10.1097/ NNE.0b013e31828dc292

Institute of Medicine. (2011). *The future of nursing: Leading change, advancing health.* http://books.nap.edu/openbook .php?record_id=12956&page=R1

International Nursing Association for Clinical Simulation and Learning Standards Committee. (2017). INACSL standards of best practice: Simulation operations. *Clinical Simulation in Nursing, 13*(12), 681–687. https://doi.org/10.1016/j .ecns.2017.10.005

Katz, J. R., Chow, C., Motzer, S. A., & Woods, S. L. (2009). The graduate record examination: Help or hindrance in nursing graduate school admissions? *Journal of Professional Nursing, 25*(6), 369–372. https://doi-org.elib.uah.edu/10.1016/j .profnurs.2009.04.002

Koivisto, J.-M., Haavisto, E., Niemi, H., Haho, P., Nylund, S., & Multisilta, J. (2018). Design principles for simulation games for learning clinical reasoning: A design-based research approach. *Nurse Education Today, 60*, 114–120. https://doi.org/10.1016/j .nedt.2017.10.002

Kopf, R. S., Watts, P. I., Meyer, E. S., & Moss, J. A. (2018). A competency-based curriculum for critical care nurse practitioners' transition to practice. *American Journal of Critical Care, 27*(5), 398–406. https://doi-org.elib.uah .edu/10.4037/ajcc2018101

LaVeist, T. A., & Pierre, G. (2014). Integrating the 3Ds — social determinants, health disparities, and health-care workforce diversity. *Public Health Reports, 129* (Suppl 2), 9–14. https:// doi: 10.1177/00333549141291S204

MacPhee, M. (2009). Developing a practice-academic partnership logic model. *Nursing Outlook, 57*, 143–147. https://doi .org//10.1016/j.outlook.2008.08.003

Marion-Martins, A. D., & Pinho, D. L. M. (2020). Interprofessional simulation effects for healthcare students: A systematic review and meta-analysis. *Nurse Education Today, 94*. https://doi.org/10.1016/j .nedt.2020.104568

McBride, A., Campbell, J., Barr, T., Duffy, J., Haozous, E., Mallow, J., Narsavage, G., Ridenour, N., & Theeke, L. (2017). The impact of the nurse faculty scholars program on schools of nursing. *Nursing Outlook, 65*(3), 327–335. Elsevier. https:// doi.org/10.1016/j.outlook.2017.01.013

Mooring, Q. E. (2016). Recruitment, advising, and retention programs — Challenges and solutions to the international problem of poor nursing student retention: A narrative literature review. *Nurse Education Today, 40*, 204–208. https://doi-org.elib.uah .edu/10.1016/j.nedt.2016.03.003

Moxley, E., Maturin, L. J., & Habtezgi, D. (2021). A lesson involving nursing management of diabetes care: Incorporating simulation in didactic instruction to prepare students for entry-level practice. *Teaching & Learning in Nursing, 16*(1), 10–15. https:// doi.org/10.1016/j.teln.2020.09.007

Mundt, M. (2018). Reflections on a dean's career: Lessons learned. *Journal of Professional Nursing, 34*(2), 142–146. http://doi.10.1016/j .profnurs.2017.07.012

Murray, T. A., Pole, D. C., Ciarlo, E. M., & Holmes, S. (2016). A nursing workforce diversity project: Strategies for recruitment, retention, graduation, and NCLEX-RN success. *Nursing Education Perspectives, 37*(3), 138–143. https://doi-org.elib.uah .edu/10.5480/14-1480

National Association of Student Personnel Administrators, Inc. (1987). *A perspective on student affairs. A statement issued on the 50th anniversary of the student personnel point of view.* https:// www.naspa.org/images/uploads/

main/A_Perspective_on_Student_
Affairs_1987.pdf

National Council of State Boards of Nursing. (2014). *NCSBN's transition to practice® study: Implications for boards of nursing.* https://www.ncsbn.org/TTP_ ImplicationsPaper_Dec2014.pdf

Njie-Carr, V. P. S., Ludeman, E., Mei C. L., Dordunoo, D., Trocky, N. M., & Jenkins, L. S. (2017). An integrative review of flipped classroom teaching models in nursing education. *Journal of Professional Nursing, 33*(2), 133–144. https://doi.org/10.1016/j .profnurs.2016.07.001

Northrup-Snyder, K., Menkens, R. M., & Ross, M. A. (2020). Can students spare the time? Estimates of online course workload. *Nurse Education Today, 90.* https://doi .org/10.1016/j.nedt.2020.104428

O'Halloran, K. C. (2019). A classification of collaboration between student and academic affairs. *College Student Journal, 53*(3), 301–314.

Phillips, J. M., & Malone, B. (2014). Increasing racial/ethnic diversity in nursing to reduce health disparities and achieve health equity. *Public Health Reports, 129*(Suppl 2), 45–50. https://doi.org/10.1177/003335491412 91S209

Pitt, V., Powis, D., Levett-Jones, T., & Hunter, S. (2014). Nursing students' personal qualities: A descriptive study. *Nurse Education Today, 34*(9), 1196–1200. https://doi-org.elib.uah .edu/10.1016/j.nedt.2014.05.004

Posey, L., Pintz, C., Zhou, Q. (Pearl), Lewis, K., & Slaven-Lee, P. (2020). Nurse practitioner student perceptions of face-to-face and telehealth standardized patient simulations. *Journal of Nursing Regulation, 10*(4), 37–44. https://doi.org/10.1016/ S2155-8256(20)30012-0

Powers, K., Neustrup, W., Thomas, C., Saine, A., Sossoman, L. B., Ferrante-Fusilli, F. A., Ross, T. C., Clark, K., & Dexter, A. (2020). Baccalaureate nursing students' experiences with multi-patient, standardized patient simulations using telehealth to collaborate. *Journal of Professional Nursing, 36*(5), 292–300. https://doi.org/10.1016/j .profnurs.2020.03.013

PR Group. (2014). *Student support redefined: 10 ways faculty can support students' success.* https://static1.squarespace.com/ static/5834c1702e69cfabd9617089/t/5a8 34cef24a69416c3e22f10/1518554351508/ Student+Support+%28Re%29defined+- +10+Ways+Everyone+Can+Support+Stude nt+Success+%28January+2014%29.pdf

Robinson-Reilly, M., Irwin, P., Coutts, R., & Slattery, N. (2020). Adding telehealth simulation into NP programs. *Nurse Practitioner, 45*(3), 44–49. https://doi .org/10.1097/01.NPR.0000653956.29721.1a

Roney, L. N., Westrick, S. J., Acri, M. C., Aronson, B. S., & Rebeschi, L. M. (2017). Technology use and technological self-efficacy among undergraduate nursing faculty. *Nursing Education Perspectives, 38*(3), 113–118. https://doi.org/10.1097/01 .NEP.0000000000000141

Scalon da Costa, L. C., Valcanti Avelino, C. C., Aparecida de Freitas, L., Machado Agostinho, A. A., Tinti de Andrade, M. B., & Takamatsu Goyatá, S. L. (2019). Undergraduates performance on vaccine administration in simulated scenario. *Revista Brasileira de Enfermagem, 72*(2), 345–353. https://doi .org/10.1590/0034-7167-2018-0486

Schuh, J. H., Biddix, J. P., Dean, L. A., & Kinzie, J. (2016). *Assessment in student affairs* (2nd ed.). John Wiley & Sons.

Skiba, D. (2017). Nursing informatics education: From automation to connected care. *Studies in Health Technology, 232,* 9–19.

Society for Simulation in Healthcare. (2020). *Accreditation.* https://www.ssih.org/ Credentialing/Accreditation

Society for Simulation in Healthcare. (2021). *Certification.* https://www.ssih.org/ Credentialing/Certification

Spector, N., Silvestre, J., Alexander, M., Martin, B., Hooper, J. I., Squires, A., & Ojemeni, M. (2020). NCSBN regulatory guidelines and evidence-based quality Indicators for nursing education programs. *Journal of Nursing Regulation, 11*(2, Supplement), S1–S64. https://doi.org/10.1016/ S2155-8256(20)30075-2

Syno, J. L. S., McBrayer, J. S., & Calhoun, D. W. (2019). Faculty and staff perceptions of organizational units and collaboration impact. *College Student Affairs Journal*, 37(1), 1–13. https://eric-ed-gov.elib .uah.edu/contentdelivery/servlet/ ERICServlet?accno=EJ1255441

Tagliareni, E. (2013). Accelerating to practice: An initiative of the NLN center for academic and practice transitions. *Nursing Education Perspectives, 34*(6), 466. https://doi.org/ 10.5480/1536-5026-34.6.430

Trepanier, S., Mainous, R., Africa, L., & Shinners, J. (2017). Nursing academic-practice partnership: The effectiveness of implementing an early residency program for nursing students. *Nurse Leader, 15*(1), 35–39. https://doi.org/10.1016/j.mnl.2016.07.010

Turner, D. M. (2020). Using high-fidelity simulation to evaluate clinical skills in prelicensure nursing students. *Nursing Education Perspectives, 41*(5), E37–E38. https://doi.org/10.1097/01 .NEP.0000000000000524

Turrise, S. L., Thompson, C. E., & Hepler, M. (2020). Virtual simulation: Comparing critical thinking and satisfaction in RN-BSN students. *Clinical Simulation in Nursing, 46*, 57–61. https://doi.org/10.1016/j.ecns.2020.03.004

Ursinus College. (2015). *Academic and student support and administrative departments: Examples of data to support institutional effectiveness*. https://www.ursinus.edu/live/ files/1441-examples-of-data-to-support-institutional

U.S. Department of Education. (2016). *Office of planning, evaluation and policy development and office of the under secretary, advancing diversity and inclusion in higher education*. https://www2.ed.gov/ rschstat/research/pubs/advancing-diversity-inclusion.pdf

U.S. Department of Health & Human Services. (2020). *What and why of usability: User experience basics*. https://www.usability. gov/what-and-why/user-experience.html

Walsh, J. A. (2020). Switching strategies: Using telehealth as an innovative virtual simulation teaching method. *Nurse Educator, 45*(6), 330. https://doi.org/10.1097/ NNE.0000000000000908

Zamanzadeh, V., Ghahramanian, A., Valizadeh, L., Bagheriyeh, F., & Lynagh, M. (2020). A scoping review of admission criteria and selection methods in nursing education. *BMC Nursing, 19*(1), 1–17. https://doi-org.elib.uah.edu/10.1186/ s12912-020-00510-1

9

Achieving Distinction Through a Commitment to Pedagogical Scholarship

Angela M. McNelis, PhD, RN, CNE, FAAN, ANEF

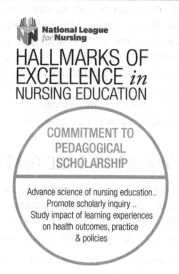

National League for Nursing

HALLMARKS OF
EXCELLENCE *in*
NURSING EDUCATION

COMMITMENT TO
PEDAGOGICAL
SCHOLARSHIP

Advance science of nursing education..
Promote scholarly inquiry ..
Study impact of learning experiences
on health outcomes, practice
& policies

INTRODUCTION

Many times people are heard to say they teach the same way they were taught. Colleagues may share concerns that their students appear unprepared for class. Fellow educators may complain that, despite how hard they work to create interesting courses and assignments, students seem disengaged. Perhaps these sentiments also describe one's own experience as a nurse educator, but one feels stuck in what to do differently. If any of these comments resonate with being a nurse educator, know that one is not alone and that evidence-based pedagogical approaches are the key to change.

Earlier chapters in this book discussed the critical importance of diverse, well-prepared faculty who enact competent teaching and contribute to a culture of continuous quality improvement in creating and sustaining learning environments that engage students. Without these essential elements, teaching and learning become stagnant and quickly fail to produce the requisite and intended outcomes. Moreover, continued use of teaching approaches that are not evidence-based, but instead are based on tradition, tacit knowledge, or professional preference (Ferguson & Day, 2005), further promote passive learning and create barriers to changing the status quo (Clapper, 2010). Pedagogical scholarship provides the evidence to guide critical aspects of learning; however, the dearth of nursing education research (Broome et al., 2012; Valiga & Ironside, 2012) and resultant data to drive teaching and evaluation of learning contribute to stagnation.

Changing the status quo requires that we use evidence-based teaching practice (EBTP) in the learning environment, just as we use evidence-based practice (EBP) in providing nursing care. To make this happen, our approach to teaching and evaluation, as well as our students' approaches to learning, must evolve. To begin, it is incumbent that we embrace the belief that creating learning environments is a mutually beneficial and collective responsibility where faculty and students come together to share knowledge, skills, and information. Then, as educators, we must first commit to critically examining our own practices and adopting EBTP strategies. Second, we must commit to becoming experts in both using and generating evidence-based pedagogies (Oermann, 2007). Finally, we must commit to facilitating student understanding of, engagement in, and contribution to using and generating evidence-based pedagogies. The *Hallmarks of Excellence in Nursing Education©* provide indicators that we can commit to addressing as we strive to attain and accomplish this transformation.

COMMITMENT TO CHANGE: USING AND GENERATING PEDAGOGY

One of the Hallmarks in this area is that faculty members and students contribute to the development of the science of nursing education through the critique, use, dissemination, and/or conduct of various forms of scholarly endeavors. Indicators faculty can use to determine if this Hallmark is being met include the following:

> To what extent do faculty members and students at all levels discuss research findings related to teaching and learning?

> In what ways do faculty members promote scholarly inquiry related to nursing education by students and colleagues?

> In what ways are faculty members and students involved in scholarly endeavors related to teaching and learning that contribute to the development of the art and science of nursing education?

Change requires critically evaluating how we teach, questioning if better approaches exist, and then using evidence as the basis for change (McCartney & Morin, 2005; Oermann, 2007); however, Patterson and Klein (2012) found some faculty did not clearly understand what is meant by evidence or EBTP. In a national survey, more than 75 percent of full-time and part-time faculty respondents considered written course evaluations as evidence, and they often confused EBTP with EBP. Similarly, Kalb et al. (2015) found that most of the 551 faculty responding to their survey valued EBTP but cited student course and faculty evaluations, as well as teaching expertise, as sources of evidence. Additionally, some indicated they were not aware of the need to use evidence in their teaching practices. These findings are concerning as they indicate faculty are not prepared to use or generate pedagogical scholarship. Lack of pedagogical knowledge prevents us from discussing research related to teaching and learning with our students and colleagues, or with potential research funders, further thwarting the development of the art and science of teaching.

The basis on which we construct courses, assignments, and activities to facilitate specific learning outcomes is not only important to us, but without such information, students have difficulty seeing the value of selected learning experiences (Fink, 2003) and may question or be dissatisfied with different approaches that require greater effort, such as teamwork and other active learning strategies. Yet, for more than 20 years, we have known active learning and cooperation among students are predictors of positive student performance and learning outcomes (Kuh et al., 1997, 2017). Dr. Marilyn Oermann explicated these critical constructs of teaching and learning in Chapter 7. Furthermore, research tells us that value, expectancy, and environment interact to produce student behaviors. Providing the rationale for course content, including materials, assignments, activities, and assessments, can provide the context, increase the value, and strengthen students' collaboration in creating a supportive and engaging learning environment (Ambrose et al., 2010; Fink, 2003; Lang, 2016). With mind, brain, and education research showing that the one who does the work does the learning (Doyle, 2008), our task as educators is to challenge students to do the work. Discussing the science for pedagogical approaches may be the key to getting student "buy-in" and engagement in different ways of learning. This context also creates a rich environment for students to contribute data on what strategies promote learning.

The research on flipped classrooms provides a good example of the positive results that can happen when students fully engage with new approaches to teaching and learning. Use of a flipped classroom has been shown to increase students' attention, engagement, and the amount and quality of time they interact with their teacher and peers (McGowan et al., 2014; McLaughlin et al., 2013). A recent study showed this approach increased knowledge of pharmacology in an accelerated bachelor of science in nursing (ABSN) program (El-Banna et al., 2017). A faculty member involved with that study shared her thoughts with this author on the effects of collaborative learning.

On the first day of the semester, when students learned we would be using a different teaching modality, we heard repeatedly, "why fix it when it's not broken." Explaining the rationale and providing research evidence for using the flipped classroom was so important, and emphasizing how this method would help them gain additional knowledge of the course material was the key to getting their buy-in. I was fortunate to be mentored by a faculty peer who had experience in this approach and was a nursing education researcher, so we both implemented and evaluated the intervention. We developed a prerecorded video that included evidence from several studies and other disciplines on the effectiveness of flipped classrooms, as well as explained the roles of student and teacher so all understood expectations for the learning environment. Students were informed this was a research study and consented to allowing us to use their quantitative data, as well as volunteered to participate in focus groups after the course to provide additional information. The results were that students who completed flipped classroom instruction had significantly higher scores on their exams and scored above the benchmark on the national criterion-referenced exam compared to students who completed the Pharmacology II course by only traditional learning strategies! This pedagogical approach is now part of the curriculum and findings were published to add to the literature.

– Malinda L. Whitlow, DNP, University of Virginia

A notable barrier to using EBTP is lack of published and rigorous research findings. The predominant use of single-group, pre- and posttest designs provide weak empirical evidence on which to guide teaching practice (Morton, 2017; Spurlock, 2018), as does the extensive use of single-site studies. The relative absence of randomized, scientifically controlled studies not only fails to contribute to an evidentiary base for EBTP, but it also reflects the paucity of funding for nursing education research (Broome et al., 2012). Although more quality research and resultant dissemination of findings has occurred during the past 10 years and there are more doctoral programs than ever before preparing students to be nursing education scholars (Ironside & Spurlock, 2014), the science of EBPT remains scant. Lack of funding makes it particularly challenging to promote scholarly inquiry related to nursing education in students and colleagues. Those who are passionate about achieving distinction, however, find paths to do this work. Several exemplars from faculty and PhD students provide narratives for working together to achieve this Hallmark, including this one from a faculty member who has emerged as a leader in building the science of nursing education.

> As a PhD student, I wanted to pursue research and scholarship in nursing education that was focused on the impact of clinical learning. As a clinician and an advanced practice registered nurse (APRN), I was aware of the importance of application of knowledge, decision-making, and clinical reasoning for safe and quality patient care. I wanted to study how to best facilitate teaching and learning of these concepts in complex care environments of today and tomorrow. I was able to find faculty mentors, despite the scarcity of faculty with this expertise, to facilitate this desire. To develop my idea of Debriefing for Meaningful Learning (DML), I used strong theoretical underpinnings and best evidence from multiple disciplines to construct and support the design of a debriefing intervention to foster clinical reasoning in nursing students. So, in very real time, I was using, constructing, and testing pedagogical approaches to improve clinical teaching and student learning.
>
> Throughout my career, I have embraced this same approach in my tripartite role of research, teaching, and service. By disseminating and incorporating my research into my teaching and service and modeling the way, I have promoted scholarly inquiry in nursing education in my bachelor's, master's, and doctoral students and advisees. Many of my students have gone on to academic careers where they are doing great work and adding to the science of nursing education. Some are pursuing new areas of inquiry including work with vulnerable students and vulnerable populations using debriefing constructs. Others are extending my work in DML. For example, some students have replicated my original study using other instruments and sample populations to grow our understanding of the development of clinical judgment and clinical decision-making in addition to clinical reasoning. Still others have used DML to study the impact with APRN students, practicing clinicians, and interdisciplinary healthcare learners, and one former student has developed and tested an instrument that measures how well DML is done. Another has developed instruments that directly test knowledge gain and application of knowledge in practice resulting from use of DML. Finally, as DML use has gone global, international students and colleagues are testing its use with different languages and educational cultures. Work with DML continues today and tomorrow, building the evidence for nursing and interdisciplinary healthcare education.
>
> – Kristina Thomas Dreifuerst, PhD, RN, CNE, FAAN,
> ANEF, Marquette University College of Nursing

As we engage in teaching, we have the option of continuing to follow traditional ways of practicing our art, or we can do something different that significantly improves the quality of student learning. The influence faculty have on promoting student scholarly inquiry cannot be underestimated and has great potential to shape the future of pedagogical scholarship in nursing, as noted by the comments a doctoral student shared with this author.

> In my role as a graduate research assistant and PhD student, I have the opportunity to work on a research team with two experienced nursing education researchers from two different institutions, as well as other temporary members of the team including researchers, faculty, and other students from around the country. The team meets weekly to discuss progress of funded research studies; however, there is also time to discuss individual educational research endeavors with feedback from experienced faculty and other team members. I contributed to the larger studies by conducting analyses and writing. I also conducted a secondary analysis of their data and, together with another PhD student, submitted a manuscript for publication! These experiences have improved my sense of inquiry as well as my data analysis and writing skills. The opportunity to work in a collaborative research team has developed my skills as a scholar through hands-on planning, implementation, evaluation, and writing. The ability to discuss current science and use that to guide research designs and educational interventions has strengthened my skills immensely and positioned me for my doctoral research as well as prepared me to launch my own program of research. I feel much more confident in the research process, nursing education scholarship, writing, and [my role] as an educator.
>
> – Sarah Beebe, MSN, CNM, WHNP-BC, CHSE,
> PhD Student & Graduate Research Assistant, The George Washington University

Simulation pedagogy perhaps provides one of the best examples of how faculty and students collaborate in scholarly endeavors that contribute to the development of the art and science of nursing education. When first adopted, simulationists had to justify its use and explain the theoretical and pedagogical foundations for why it would work as an educational intervention. These pioneers had to rigorously design and evaluate each aspect of the simulation, including student learning outcomes, to get "buy-in" from colleagues. Student engagement and willingness to participate in evaluation was paramount to establishing the use and validity of the strategy (S. Kardong-Edgren, personal communication, October 8, 2020). A faculty member and leader in the International Association of Clinical Simulation and Learning shared with this author an example of faculty and students working together to co-create an effective learning experience for students.

> After reviewing simulation content across the curriculum, the decision was made to create a simulation that focused on community health. We went to the National League for Nursing (NLN) Advancing Care Excelled Series (ACES) cases and chose the Julia Morales and Lucy Grey case to use as a foundation. We altered the case so that the three key roles in the case were two young males in a same-sex relationship, and the mother of the dying patient. In this simulation, Joseph, a 25-year-old Hispanic male, was dying of cancer and had not communicated with [his] father in years. The learning objectives were on discussing entry into hospice, communicating end-of-life wishes, and delivering culturally sensitive care to a same-sex couple. We piloted the new simulation by enlisting volunteer students to play

the student roles. We provided them with the planned preparation material that included readings on end-of-life conversations, [learning about] hospice, and providing culturally appropriate care to same-sex couples. We ran the simulation one time, and then did a joint debriefing with students, faculty, and standardized patients (SPs) to identify if the simulation met the identified objectives, had the appropriate background information and script for the SPs, and, among other items, if the prebriefing materials adequately prepared the students for the simulation. After this debriefing, we make identified corrections and run through the simulation again, this time doing a traditional debriefing. The students and the SPs were equal partners with the faculty in making the determination on the final product.

In the initial debriefing after the first pilot of this simulation, we realized we had made a mistake! We had prepared for a debriefing about end of life and same-sex couples. What we found was that the students were entirely comfortable with the concept of caring for a same-sex couple. What they were not comfortable with was the lack of support from the father. Their stress in the simulation came from managing communication issues with the parents. This was not the direction that the faculty planned for but did represent a key learning opportunity for students. We changed the preparatory materials and debriefing guide to reflect the true learning that occurred in the simulation. Without incorporating the students as partners in the evaluation of the pilot simulation, we would not have had such a clear picture of the power of this simulation.

– Carla Nye, DNP, CPNP-BC, CNE, CHSE,
Virginia Commonwealth University School of Nursing

As discussed extensively in Chapter 11, the NLN (2020a) Centers of Excellence in Nursing Education™ designation for schools/colleges of nursing use criteria that are consistent with the Hallmarks, and many criteria are closely aligned with the Hallmark being explored here. Similarly, the NLN Core Competencies of Nurse Educators©, used to guide the development of the Certified Nurse Educator (CNE) exam, include a role expectation of engaging in scholarship that focuses on understanding and using EBTPs or engaging in the scholarship of teaching (Christensen & Simmons, 2020; NLN, 2020b). Yet, a recent study assessing these competencies in a national sample of 529 masters of science in nursing education or post-master's certificate programs found that less than half of the programs' course descriptions included engaging in scholarship as a programmatic outcome (Fitzgerald et al., 2020). Additionally, few programs required both use and generation of scholarly work. Despite many schools achieving COE distinction and many faculty achieving CNE status, the evidentiary base for teaching practices in nursing remains limited. While the current state of the science is disappointing, the NLN is resolute in changing the paradigm. Professional development, research funding, recognition, and certification all are testaments to the priority the organization makes to achieving excellence and distinction through pedagogical scholarship.

COMMITMENT TO CHANGE: LINKING STUDENT LEARNING TO HEALTH OUTCOMES

Another Hallmark is that faculty members and students explore the influence of student learning experiences on the health of the individuals and populations they serve in various healthcare settings. Attainment of this Hallmark can be assessed by considering the following indicators:

▸ What strategies are used to systematically document the extent to which student learning experiences affect healthcare outcomes for the populations they serve?

▸ To what extent do leaders in partner healthcare facilities report improved patient care outcomes or more effective nursing practices in areas where students have extended learning experiences?

▸ To what extent do student learning experiences influence nursing practice and/or healthcare policies?

Although some progress has been made toward realizing this Hallmark, relatively little published evidence exists to document scholarly work in this area. Just as there are difficulties encountered in studying educational interventions in the academic setting, studying the connection between student learning experiences and patient outcomes also has significant challenges and is complicated, as many extraneous variables affect outcomes. For example, lack of consistency and/or frequency of student placement, as well as variability in level of participation in patient care (McNelis et al., 2014), makes it nearly impossible to connect student experiences with patient outcomes. Moreover, studying the connection necessitates evaluating student learning, which historically has been a substantial problem for nurse educators. Valiga and Ironside (2012) noted that many studies use easily measured outcomes such as student satisfaction or confidence rather than outcomes linked to the learning objectives. Similarly and more recently, in a systematic review of pre-licensure nursing student learning in traditional clinical experiences, no quantitative studies were found with rigorous methodologies, including valid and reliable outcome measures, despite no year restrictions on the search (Leighton et al., 2021). Thus, if student learning cannot be objectively measured, how can a link to patient care be determined? The Hallmarks challenge us to move our profession forward to address these indicators and reach for excellence.

The doctor of nursing practice (DNP) prepares nurses to function in complex healthcare environments using scientific knowledge and practice expertise to assure quality patient outcomes (American Association of Colleges of Nursing [AACN], 2006). DNP-prepared nurses implement and evaluate the science developed by other researchers to improve patient care. Thus, one of the major deliverables of DNP programs is the final project that focuses on implementing a change to improve healthcare outcomes. As educators mentoring DNP students, we support student use of EBP and quality improvement tools to develop and implement their projects. Additionally, we are positioned to facilitate dissemination of their work to document the link between student learning experiences and health outcomes. Comments shared with this author by the director of DNP scholarly projects at one school reflect how student projects have been linked to patient outcomes; perhaps the time has come to consider documenting the connections between health outcomes and the care provided by students in other programs as well.

As the director of scholarly projects for the DNP, I work with DNP faculty mentors to successfully engage students in learning experiences that demonstrate positive nursing practice and/or policy outcomes by aligning student projects with the strategic aims of the practice organization. DNP projects that are planned, implemented, and evaluated with a team of faculty and practice partners demonstrate improvement in patient outcomes and sustained success. I share two exemplary projects that connect student learning with improvement in care.

A new handoff communication tool was used to improve the safety culture of the nurses in the pre-op and operating room (OR) units. The IOWA Model of EBP translation was used to guide the DNP project. Faculty mentored the student in a critical appraisal and synthesis of the literature to locate an evidence-based handoff tool appropriate for implementation at the practice site. The DNP student collaborated with practice leaders and educators to implement an education plan for staff. Nursing staff were surveyed before and after the education on the handoff communication tool regarding the culture of safety on their units. The results of the survey revealed a statistically significant improvement in the perception of safety culture for nurses in the pre-op and OR units as measured by the handoff transition and patient safety scores. It is important to note that 100 percent of respondents gave their unit a safety grade of acceptable or higher on the post-survey. To sustain this practice change, the handoff communication tool was embedded in the electronic health record, unit policies were updated, and annual monitoring to collect and review future safety culture survey results were implemented.

The second example is a project focused on critically ill patients. Research shows that sleep deprivation caused by frequent nighttime interruptions is associated with poor sleep quality and negative patient outcomes. In consultation and collaboration with the DNP student, the practice site identified the need to improve sleep quality and decrease the incidence of intensive care unit (ICU) delirium. Faculty guided the DNP student to implement a quality improvement project to promote uninterrupted sleep between the hours of 10 p.m. and 5 a.m. for eligible patients in the ICU. This evidence-based, nurse-driven, nonpharmacological implementation of an ICU sleep checklist contained nine interventions to reduce noise, light, and iatrogenic sleep disturbances. The protocol is safe, inexpensive, and easy to implement. Findings showed improvement in the rate of ICU delirium, and suggest that by promoting sleep, ICU nurses can prevent the onset of delirium. Sustainability of the practice change was secured by embedding the sleep quality assessment into the electronic health record.

– Karen Kesten, DNP, APRN, CCNS, CNE, CCRN-K, FAAN,
The George Washington University School of Nursing

DNP projects, such as those previously described, illustrate the critical need for partnership between academia and practice in advancing pedagogical scholarship. Engaging stakeholders and clinical partners to develop, implement, evaluate, and disseminate a project that addresses a significant problem creates meaningful learning experiences (Buckley et al., 2020). The partnership also provides an opportunity for identification of salient patient care outcome indicators. Collaborations with healthcare organizations strengthen the value of such projects and further our efforts to bridge the gap between academia and practice, and document the positive impact each can have on the other. Additionally, leaders in academia and healthcare organizations should work together to create cultures where resources, policies, and processes are shared to support learning environments (Irby, 2018), as reflected in these comments shared with this author by a former chief nursing officer (CNO).

In my decade as a chief nurse, I never had a school of nursing academic program come to me with any sort of request to evaluate the patient outcomes related to the student learning experience – it was always more of an evaluation of the student experiences or our partnership activities. We should be so bold as to make a recommendation to national nursing organizations who publish guidelines on practice partnership standards to include more outcomes evaluation of the clinical impact of student contributions. The idea of CNOs and academic deans working together to create an evaluation of the OUTCOMES of the student contribution (at the undergraduate and graduate level) to patient care is needed. Quite frankly, I feel like CNOs would be so responsive and it would help to encourage more of a learning partnership in practice. With quantifiable outcomes of student impact on patients, it would most likely increase clinical experiences for students as well.

– Karen Drenkard, PhD, RN, NEA-BC, FAAN,
The George Washington University School of Nursing

The NLN (2020a) champions the idea of creating partnerships as shown by its newest Center of Excellence designation, "Creating Workplace Environments that Promote the Academic Progression of Nurses," that is awarded to healthcare organizations. One criterion for this designation is that academic/practice partnerships yield projects to advance evidence-based nursing practice. Similarly, recognizing the importance of academic-practice partnerships, the American Association of Colleges of Nursing-American Organization of Nurse Executives (AACN-AONE) Task Force on Academic-Practice Partnerships (2012) developed eight guiding principles for improving the health of the population through effective care delivery systems. These guiding principles include a focus on mutual goals with set evaluation periods; commitment to lifelong learning; shared knowledge of current best practices; joint research and funding to design, implement, and sustain innovative patient-centered delivery systems; and analysis of workforce and education data (see AACN-AONE Task Force on Academic-Practice Partnerships, 2012 for a full description). Clearly, they align with the NLN Hallmarks to provide clear direction to academic institutions and healthcare organizations for advancing nursing practice to improve the health of the public.

To further address the Hallmarks and achieve distinction, an additional principle is proposed: Partners work to quantify the contribution of nursing students (at every level — undergraduate, graduate, and doctoral) to the outcomes of patient care. This includes co-creating the metrics, collecting and evaluating data, and disseminating findings across academic and practice settings. It is only with this level of rigorous pedagogical scholarship that we can generate evidence to drive nursing practice in local, national, and global healthcare settings, as well as policies that guide our profession.

A recent global project illustrates the power and ingenuity of faculty, students, and healthcare partners working together to address a significant community health issue. Working with colleagues in Haiti, the faculty and students noted here discussed how they developed, implemented, and evaluated a sustainable intervention to address childhood anemia.

Our research team, including nursing students, conducted a study to investigate factors associated with childhood anemia. We explored perspectives, understanding, and ideas for solutions from community members in Haiti. Participants were children aged 6 months to 14 years, their families, and any community members attending the free clinic. Student nurses were integral to the healthcare team, collecting health data, providing health education, and participating in focus groups. The study found a high prevalence of childhood anemia and an overall low level of understanding of multiple causes of anemia. Community members were committed and willing to make changes necessary to improve childhood anemia in their community and continued the educational intervention in their community. Findings also informed the plan for a follow-up study using a community-based action plan that employed evidence-based teaching and learning activities, including the development of an animated educational video on childhood anemia to increase children and parents' knowledge about anemia prevention.

– Joyce Pulcini, PhD, PNP-BC, FAAN, FAANP; Jeongyoung Park, PhD;
Carol S. Lang, DScN, MScN, RN, and Mayri Leslie, EdD,
MSN, CNM, FACNM, The George Washington University School of Nursing

A final example of partnership is the dedicated education unit (DEU), an academic-practice collaborative clinical learning model. This synergistic educational environment is created through committed leadership, active engagement of clinically expert staff, and academically expert faculty embedded in mentoring and teaching students (Glazer et al., 2011; Moscato et al., 2007). Used predominantly at the pre-licensure level, the model could be enhanced by leveraging research expertise and data from electronic health record systems to identify and systematically document the impact of student learning experiences on patient outcomes (Pryse et al., 2020).

CONCLUSION

Benner and colleagues (2010) identified the need to support ongoing faculty growth in pedagogy for those educating students as a prerequisite for improvement in the quality of their teaching. However, when faculty lack awareness and skills to enact EBTP, they continue to teach as they were taught and fail to contribute to the science of nursing education scholarship. Our commitment and responsibility to prepare the next generation of nurses must also include modeling best practices in teaching and learning with pre-licensure and graduate students. A final exemplar, co-created by a former faculty member and her mentee, and shared with this author, illustrates the power of faculty "planting the seeds" of EBTP and engaging students in scholarship. Relationships such as these are key to preparing the next generation of scholars who will create needed change.

From a former faculty member: From student to colleague describes my journey of engaging in collaborative scholarly inquiry in the art and science of nursing. I met Kathleen nine years ago when she was a student on the first-ever credit-toward-major global clinical in a California public school of nursing. I knew Kathleen to be a bright and conscientious student who was reserved and quiet in group settings, and early on I asked about her short-and long-term goals as a nurse. She identified a desire to continue her education into graduate school and I offered to serve as her mentor. There are several factors I believe led to her successful journey through undergraduate and graduate degrees and to her present status as a PhD student committed to working in global health education and policy. First, I included her in all aspects of my research in global service learning, providing the pedagogical underpinnings for this learning approach. Second, I included her on my research team. There were starts and stops as Kathleen began to increase her responsibilities within the team, but we constantly discussed progress and identified next steps. We have now collaborated for nearly 10 years and she has transitioned from student to colleague. I believe acknowledgement of contributions and celebration of accomplishments is important and including Kathleen as a co-author in the team's publications helped to increase her confidence as a scholar as well as her commitment to the scholarship of nursing education.

– Tamara McKinnon, RN, DNP, APHN,
FAAN, Global Wellsprings/Cultural Mindfulness Consulting

From the former faculty member's mentee: Before I met Dr. McKinnon I had been involved in campus programs related to global health education, but I often found myself standing as the only nursing student in the room. I was interested in incorporating these interests in my nursing career and graduate school but didn't know (or believe) if I could get there. In my final year of nursing school, I met Dr. McKinnon and was inspired by her work and passion for global health. She took me under her wing soon thereafter. I soon found myself supporting Dr. McKinnon with her research and presentations, taking every opportunity to learn from her. She also invited me to join an exceptional research team, and over the years, I have come to see members of that team as mentors as well. Things seemed to come full circle a few years later when I found myself with Dr. McKinnon co-leading the same faculty-led program in Ireland I had attended as her student. I observed Dr. McKinnon's use of evidence-based teaching with the students, modeling behaviors and skills, and finally stepping aside so they could take the lead. Throughout the program, the students flourished, making their own connections and engaging with our partners in Ireland. Because of Dr. McKinnon's mentorship, I am currently a doctoral nursing student conducting dissertation research in global health. I now find myself exploring this area of research in a way I had only dreamt of while in nursing school. As I consider my future after graduation, I aim to continue this research as a nurse educator and generate evidence to drive teaching and guide nursing policy and regulation.

– Kathleen de Leon, MS, RN, PhD Student,
University of California San Francisco

Bass (1999) identified and summarized a foundational issue in teaching more than two decades ago, but one that continues to impact nursing and our commitment to pedagogical scholarship today. Research is driven by a problem, yet in teaching, we do not want to have a problem. He posited that "changing the status of the problem in teaching from terminal remediation to ongoing investigation is precisely what the movement for a scholarship of teaching is all about" (p. 1). Transformation requires that we reframe our teaching as a problem that needs to be examined and potentially changed. Reframing allows for professional growth as well as provides the foundation for scholarship, dissemination, and improved student learning.

This chapter was written during the COVID-19 pandemic, a great crisis impacting every aspect of our lives, including aspects of nursing education, and causing many problems. The interruption and disruption in how we taught and how students learned forced drastic and rapid changes, many just "bandages to stop the bleeding" rather than strategies guided by evidence. As educators, we can use this time and place as an opportunity to commit (or recommit) to pedagogical scholarship to address problems by using and generating EBTPs.

References

Ambrose, S. A., Bridges, M. W., DiPietro, M., Lovett, M. C., & Norman, M. K. (2010). *How learning works: Seven research-based principles for smart teaching.* John Wiley & Sons.

American Association of Colleges of Nursing. (2006). *The essentials of doctoral education for advanced nursing practice.* https://www.aacnnursing.org/Portals/42/Publications/DNPEssentials.pdf

American Association of Colleges of Nursing-American Organization of Nurse Executives Task Force on Academic-Practice Partnerships. (2012). *Guiding principles to academic-practice partnership.* American Association of Colleges of Nursing. https://www.aacnnursing.org/Academic-Practice-Partnerships/The-Guiding-Principles

Bass, R. (1999). The scholarship of teaching: What's the problem? *Inventio, 1*(1). https://sotl.gmu.edu/wp-content/uploads/2019/03/Bass-SOTL-article-1998.pdf

Benner, P., Sutphen, M., Leonard, V., & Day, L. (2010). *Educating nurses: A call for radical transformation.* Jossey-Bass.

Broome, M. E., Ironside, P. M., & McNelis, A. M. (2012). Research in nursing education: State of the science. *Journal of Nursing Education, 51,* 521–524. https://doi.org/10.3928/01484834-20120820-10

Buckley, K. M., Idzik, S., Bingham, D., Windemuth, B., & Bindonet, S. L. (2020). Structuring doctor of nursing practice project courses to facilitate success and ensure rigor. *Journal of Professional Nursing, 36*(4), 206–211. https://doi.org/10.1016/j.profnurs.2019.12.001

Christensen, L. S., & Simmons, L. E. (2020). *The scope of practice for academic nurse educators and academic clinical nurse educators* (3rd ed.). National League for Nursing.

Clapper, T. C. (2010). Beyond Knowles: What those conducting simulation need to know about adult learning theory? *Clinical Simulation in Nursing, 6*(1), e7–e14. https://doi.org/10.1016/j.ecns.2009.07.003

Doyle, T. (2008). *Helping students learn in a learner-centered environment: A guide to facilitating learning in higher education.* Stylus Publishing, LLC.

El-Banna, M. M., Whitlow, M., & McNelis, A. M. (2017). Flipping around the classroom: Accelerated bachelor of science in nursing students' satisfaction and achievement. *Nurse Education Today, 56,* 41–46. https://doi.org/10.1016/j.nedt.2017.06.003

Ferguson, L., & Day, R. (2005). Evidence-based nursing education: Myth or reality? *The Journal of Nursing Education, 44*(3), 107–115. https://doi.org/10.3928/01484834-20050301-03

Fink, L. D. (2003). *Creating significant learning experiences: An integrated approach to designing college courses.* John Wiley & Sons.

Fitzgerald, A., McNelis, A. M., & Billings, D. M. (2020). NLN core competencies for nurse educators: Are they present in the course descriptions of Academic Nurse Educator programs? *Nursing Education Perspectives, 41*(1), 4–9. https://doi.org/10.1097/01.NEP.0000000000000530

Glazer, G., Ives Erickson, J., Mylott, L., Mulready-Shick, J., & Banister, G. (2011). Partnering and leadership: Core requirements for developing a dedicated education unit. *The Journal of Nursing Administration, 41*(10), 401–406. https://doi.org/10.1097/NNA.0b013e31822edd79

Irby, D. M. (2018). Improving environments for learning in the health professions. In *Proceedings of a conference sponsored by Josiah Macy Jr. Foundation in April.* Joseph Macy Jr. Foundation. https://macyfoundation.org/assets/reports/publications/macy_monograph_2018_webfile.pdf

Ironside, P. M., & Spurlock, D. R. (2014). Getting serious about building nursing education science. *Journal of Nursing Education, 53*(12), 667–669. https://doi.org/10.3928/01484834-20141118-10

Kalb, K. A., O'Conner-Von, S. K., Brockway, C., Rierson, C. L., & Sendelbach, S. (2015).

Evidence-based teaching practice in nursing education: Faculty perspectives and practices. *Nursing Education Perspectives*, 36(4), 212–219. https://doi.org/10.5480/14-1472

Kuh, G., O'Donnell, K., & Schneider, C. (2017). HIPs at ten. *Change: The Magazine of Higher Learning, 49*(5), 8–16. https://doi.org/10.1080/00091383.2017.1366805

Kuh, G. D., Pace, C. R., & Vesper, N. (1997). The development of process indicators to estimate student gains associated with good practices in undergraduate education. *Research in Higher Education, 38*(4), 435–454. https://doi.org/10.1023/A:1024962526492

Lang, J. M. (2016). *Small teaching: Everyday lessons from the science of learning*. Jossey-Bass.

Leighton, K., Kardong-Edgren, S., McNelis, A. M., Foisy-Doll, C., & Sullo, E. (2021). Objective outcomes of traditional clinical experiences in prelicensure nursing education: An empty systematic review. *Journal of Nursing Education, 60*(3), 136–142. https://doi.org/10.3928/01484834-20210222-03

McCartney, P., & Morin, K. (2005). Where is the evidence for teaching methods used in nursing education? *MCN. The American Journal of Maternal Child Nursing, 30*(6), 406–412. https://doi.org/10.1097/00005721-200511000-00010

McGowan, B. S., Balmer, J. T., & Chappell, K. (2014). Flipping the classroom: A data-driven model for nursing education. *Journal of Continuing Education in Nursing, 45*(11), 477–488. https://doi.org/10.3928/00220124-20141027-11

McLaughlin, J., Griffin, L., Esserman, D., Davidson, C., Glatt, D., Roth, M., Gharkholonarehe, N., & Mumper, R. (2013). Pharmacy student engagement, performance, and perception in a flipped satellite classroom. *American Journal of Pharmaceutical Education, 77*(9), 196–196. https://doi.org/10.5688/ajpe779196

McNelis, A. M., Ironside, P. M., Ebright, P. R., Dreifuerst, K. T., Zvonar, S. E., & Conner, S. C. (2014). Learning nursing practice: A multisite, multimethod investigation of clinical education. *Journal of Nursing Regulation, 4*(4), 30–35. https://doi.org/10.1016/S2155-8256(15)30115-0

Morton, P. G. (2017). Nursing education research: An editor's view. *Journal of Professional Nursing, 33*(5), 311–312. https://doi.org/10.1016/j.profnurs.2017.08.002

Moscato, S. R., Miller, J., Logsdon, K., Weinberg, S., & Chorpenning, L. (2007). Dedicated education unit: An innovative clinical partner education model. *Nursing Outlook, 55*(1), 31–37. https://doi.org/10.1016/j.outlook.2006.11.001

National League for Nursing. (2020a). *Center of Excellence in Nursing Education applicant handbook*. http://www.nln.org/docs/default-source/default-document-library/2021-coe-handbook.pdf?sfvrsn=0

National League for Nursing. (2020b). *Certified Nurse Educator (CNE®) 2020 candidate handbook*. http://www.nln.org/docs/default-source/default-document-library/cne-handbook-sept-2020.pdf?sfvrsn=2

Oermann, M. H. (2007). Approaches to gathering evidence for educational practices in nursing. *The Journal of Continuing Education in Nursing, 38*(6), 250–255; quiz 256–257, 270. https://doi.org/10.3928/00220124-20071101-05

Patterson, B., & Klein, J. (2012). Evidence for teaching: What are faculty using? *Nursing Education Perspectives, 33*(4), 240–245. https://doi.org/10.5480/1536-5026-33.4.240

Pryse, Y. M., Heiskell, J., Goetz, J., Hittle, B. M., & Glazer, G. (2020). Dedicated education units: Redirecting for success. *Nurse Education in Practice, 46,* 102806. https://doi.org/10.1016/j.nepr.2020.102806

Spurlock, D. R. (2018). The single-group, pre- and posttest design in nursing education research: It's time to move on. *Journal of Nursing Education, 57*(2), 69–71. https://doi.org/10.3928/01484834-20180123-02

Valiga, T. M., & Ironside, P. M. (2012). Crafting a national agenda for nursing education research. *Journal of Nursing Education, 51*(1), 3–6. https://doi.org/10.3928/01484834-20111213-01

10

Effective Institutional and Professional Leadership: Essential to Achieve Excellence and Distinction in Nursing Education

Demetrius James Porche, DNS, PhD, PCC, FACHE, FAANP, FAAN, ANEF

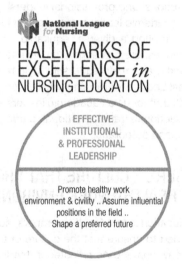

National League *for* **Nursing**

HALLMARKS OF EXCELLENCE *in* NURSING EDUCATION

EFFECTIVE INSTITUTIONAL & PROFESSIONAL LEADERSHIP

Promote healthy work environment & civility .. Assume influential positions in the field .. Shape a preferred future

INTRODUCTION

Effective institutional and professional leadership in academia is essential to provide the environment, culture, and expectations that are essential to achieve excellence and distinction in nursing education. Distinctive leaders and leadership require a differentiation that is "notable." Effective institutional and professional leadership that is excellent is considered more than an outcome. Excellence in leadership is actually a journey of continual pursuit toward something that creates a status of recognition as being "notable or set apart from others" – in other words, distinctive – and as this book asserts, that "something" is excellence in nursing education. Effective leadership is visionary, mission focused, inspires others to pursue excellence, and promotes a positive and healthy organizational culture and climate, while cultivating a culture of innovation. Leadership is also addressed in Chapter 3 on engaged students as students commit to a professional nursing role and in Chapter 4 on diverse, well-prepared faculty where the faculty complement is composed of nurse leaders who have expertise in areas of practice, education, and/or research.

LEADERSHIP STYLES

Leadership is a vogue and popular concept that seems simple with many academics expressing a desire to be leaders, but few of them being willing to take on the challenges of a formal leadership position. Some academics want to be leaders, not managers; others desire to engage in transformational leadership but not transactional leadership. Few would argue the fact, however, that effective leadership is a complex, dynamic role that includes managing while leading with the ability to exhibit multiple leadership styles, sometimes in the same situation – being both transactional and transformational, for example. Effective institutional and professional leadership in an academic environment necessitates that the academic leader remain mission focused, outcomes driven, and values based while promoting a diverse, equitable, and inclusive organizational culture and climate. Effective leaders can engage in diverse organizational and professional environmental contexts, and their leadership style reflects fluidity. This chapter addresses the three National League for Nursing (NLN) *Hallmarks of Excellence in Nursing Education*© (NLN, 2020) that focus on academic leaders and leadership, embracing all leadership styles – transactional, transformational, participative, collaborative, servant, bureaucratic, strategic, and autocratic.

LEADERSHIP TO ENSURE A CULTURE THAT PROMOTES EXCELLENCE AND A HEALTHY WORK ENVIRONMENT

One Hallmark in nursing education is that faculty members, administrators, and students provide the leadership needed to ensure that the culture of the school promotes excellence and a healthy work environment. As reflected in the Indicators for this Hallmark, such a culture and healthy environment is characterized by *collegial dialogue*, particularly about positive teaching/learning environments and the responsibility of faculty and students in the creation of a positive teaching/learning environment; *collaboration* that creates learning environments that empower diverse student populations; *creativity and innovation* in designing and implementing programs that prepare graduates for a volatile, uncertain, complex, and ambiguous (VUCA) healthcare environment; and *safety, ethical behavior, civility, and collegiality*. Central tenets of this Hallmark are organizational culture and climate, innovation, change management, and embracing excellence.

Culture and Climate

Schein (2016) describes organizational culture as the underlying beliefs, assumptions, values, and manner of interacting within an organization. An organizational climate is the shared perceptions of members of the institution and profession and is the way the faculty, staff, and students experience the academic environment. Effective leaders are responsible for promoting an organizational culture and climate that supports collegial dialogue, innovation, change, creativity, values, and ethical behavior. It is often said that "culture eats strategy for lunch."

Three critical aspects of a culture that effective leaders must attend to are observable artifacts, espoused values, and basic assumptions. Some *visible artifacts* in an academic environment are signage, images of nurses, presence of mission, values, and ethical and/or professional standards displayed, along with interior architectural design elements. *Espoused values* are the institution's or profession's expressed core values, which effective leaders collaborate with others to fully integrate into the fiber of the organizational culture and climate. The core values, in addition to the mission, vision, and goals, become the lens by which academic decisions are rendered, and they are evidenced by behaviors that are ethical and research- or evidence-based. The *assumptions* are the often unconscious determinants of an institution's thought processes and actions. Effective leaders should illuminate the underlying assumptions and be attentive to how unconscious biases impact the creation and sustaining of a diverse, equitable, and inclusive academic environment. Effective leaders promote a climate of memorable or defining moments such as achieving national recognition for accomplishments or recognizing faculty or students publicly for displaying the institution's core values. These moments elevate faculty, staff, and students above the everyday mundane activities, provide an insightful burst of revelation and understanding, promote a sense of pride about individual and institutional achievements, and promote social moments of connection and interaction (Heath & Health, 2017).

Coyle (2018) proposes creating a culture code that requires cohesion and cooperation among a diverse population of faculty, staff, and students to "function with a single mindset" to achieve the academic mission. The culture code proposes that effective leaders build a safe environment that supports constructive and inclusive dialogue in an atmosphere of fun, creativity and innovation, and mutual support. This safe environment is considered the glue that creates a sense of organizational belonging. The sense of belonging opens a culture and climate in which academicians can share their vulnerabilities and translate these into a sense of connection and trusting cooperation to achieve a level of distinction that may be a risky venture. Sharing of personal life experience and feelings promotes a sense of belonging but could create a feeling of personal vulnerability or fear. Lastly, Coyle emphasizes that an established clear purpose (mission) is necessary as a component of the culture code.

Effective leaders know that the success of the academic unit is dependent on the culture. Academic leaders should strive to create a contagious positive organizational culture and climate. Cavanaugh (2020) reminds leaders that leadership influence is also about using oneself as a leadership instrument. The leader should infect the academic unit with positive culture. A contagious culture is about intentionality, energy, and executive presence (discussed later). As leaders engage their sphere of influence in the academic environment, nursing profession, and community, the leader should be intentional about who and what they want to infect (Cavanaugh, 2016).

Innovation

Academic institutions are ripe with traditions, but effective leaders promote innovation so that new, unique, and distinct methods, products, goods, or services are created.

Gibson (2015) proposes four innovation lenses academic leaders can use to promote innovation and elicit generative and creative thinking: challenging orthodoxies, harnessing trends, leveraging resources, and understanding needs.

Challenging orthodoxies involves calling the status quo and traditional paradigms into question, and it requires the proposal of sometimes wild and antithetical alternative solutions as a means to fundamentally drive innovative change. Being aware of and understanding the variety of trends occurring in nursing practice, nursing education, and higher education — as revealed through continuous environmental scanning — allows the effective leader to identify disruptive opportunities for change. Although academic institutions are frequently stressed with limited resources, effective academic leaders need to *leverage those resources* to encourage faculty, staff, and students to adopt a mindset where they see themselves as capable of generating and implementing new and innovative ideas for transformational change. Lastly, the lens of *understanding needs* ensures alignment of the innovation to the needed area of change; change for the sake of change alone can have a negative influence on cultural climate. Innovative change should be needs- and evidence-based (Gibson, 2015).

Change

Innovation necessitates change management, which often is a challenge for academic leaders who exist within environments that are rich in symbolism, rituals, and traditions. As academic leaders propose innovative changes, there is a definite possibility that fear will lead to change resistance. Proposed change needs to be research/evidence-based, align with the expressed vision and mission of the organization, embrace the core values, and planned in a way that integrates change champions and motivate laggards in order to enhance success.

Change management can be achieved in eight steps as outlined by Kotter and Cohen (2002). The following steps make up this decisive structure for effective change:

1. Create the sense of a burning bridge or urgency that presents a compelling emotional and business case for the needed change.

2. Stack the team with powerful and influential members who are supportive champions and charismatic enough to create a desire to follow and change.

3. Create a clear, simple, and motivational vision for change that outlines specific strategies needed for change execution.

4. Communicate a simple, heart-felt message using multiple communication channels and mediums about the need for the change, change process, status of the change, and expected and actual outcomes of the change.

5. Empower faculty, staff, and students to engage in the change process while removing obstacles and barriers to change.

6. Strategically plan the implementation of the change to signal the accomplishment of short-term outcomes.

7. Execute an executive presence that maintains momentum during the change process.

8. Integrate the change into the academic institutional culture and climate.

The effective academic leader who follows these steps is likely to be successful in leading and managing the changes that may be needed to achieve excellence in nursing education and achieve distinction for the school's students, faculty, and staff.

Embracing Excellence

A culture of excellence promotes the attraction and retention of exemplary faculty, staff, and students to the academic unit. An academic culture that embraces excellence is committed to a clear vision, mission, and values that supports innovation in an environment of trust and respect. A culture of excellence should be a "way of academic life" with the continual pursuit of and quest for knowledge generation. Ashby and Pell (2001) propose 10 features of "great" organizational cultures: missionary zeal; sense of pride, sincerity, and cooperation; attitude of constructive discontent; value-based mindset and management style; emphasis on creativity and innovation; commitment to develop role models and leaders; sense of high expectations and professional standards; fair, commensurate compensation and incentive program; habit of celebrating successes; and adhering to the golden rule — "do unto others as you would have them do unto you."

Academic institutions embracing excellence must hire qualified and committed faculty and staff and admit qualified students who are motivated to learn. They also must ensure that the values and professional goals of faculty, staff, and students are aligned with the academic institution's vision and mission and ensure that the right individuals are doing the right jobs, with the right teams, in the right environments, and with the right resources. Successful on-boarding of faculty, staff, and students is critical to ensuring the academic institution's expectations are known and academic culture and climate remain intact.

FACULTY, ADMINISTRATORS, STUDENTS, AND ALUMNI ARE RESPECTED AS LEADERS

A second Hallmark related to institutional and professional leadership is that faculty members, administrators, students, and alumni are respected as leaders in the parent institution, as well as in local, state, regional, national, and/or international communities. Indicators that this Hallmark has been achieved include the following: faculty and administrators hold influential leadership positions on institutional committees, task forces, policy-making groups, and other similar bodies; students hold influential positions on school/college or institutional committees, task forces, or other bodies; faculty members and administrators are appointed to, elected to, or serve on boards, institutes, or other similar bodies; and the work of faculty, administrators, and students influence systemic change in the nursing profession and healthcare system. Academic leaders who create environments where outcomes such as these can be achieved exude a sense of executive presence, maintain an open mindset, and demonstrate emotional intelligence.

Executive Presence

What is executive presence? While it may be somewhat difficult to define succinctly, it is something we know when we see and feel it. It is the person who walks into the room exuding confidence and credibility or the person who seems to command a room or have the ability to astutely ingratiate the entire room with their being.

One might question whether executive presence is important for nursing, and the answer to that question would be a resounding "Yes!" The nursing profession has long desired to be "at the decision-making table or in the board room," and concerned with the "image of nursing"; however, this has to be achieved through presence, specifically executive presence. Academic leaders have the potential to demonstrate executive presence within the nursing unit, within the broader academic institution, and within the local, state, regional, and national nursing communities.

Executive presence, which co-exists with authentic leadership, is considered as an essential component of effective leadership. A leader with executive presence has a combination of confidence, poise, and authenticity that convinces others that they are in the presence of someone who is "the real deal." Executive presence is not a performance measure but a measure of image, and it can be thought of as the dynamic combination of three executive presence pillars: gravitas, communication, and appearance (Hewlett, 2016).

Gravitas is about how a leader acts. It is the core characteristic of executive presence and the pillar that represents the domain of knowledge. A leader who is characterized by gravitas has the ability to go at least six questions deep in a nursing or academic knowledge domain. A gravitas leader convinces others that they have the knowledge and ability to be entrusted with serious academic responsibility. The six key behaviors of gravitas are confidence and grace under fire, decisiveness with difficult decisions, integrity and veracity (speaking truth to power), reputation precedence or personal leadership brand that is respected, a focused vision, and emotional intelligence (Hewlett, 2016).

The second pillar of executive presence is *communication*. Leaders with executive presence are expected to have a mastery of verbal and nonverbal communication skills, an understanding of the complexity of the communication process, and a commitment to the critical element of communication – "listening." Leaders with executive presence ensure that they listen to others and that others hear and feel their communication. Consistent with Maya Angelou's quote, "People will forget what you said, people will forget what you did, but people will never forget how you made them feel," communication with executive presence is not so much about "what" is said, but rather about "how" it is said. Some characteristics of communication in executive presence are the ability to command a room, establish a connection, deliver words in a succinct manner with a fluid pace, use narratives and storytelling, demonstrate direct and assertive communication, read a room, and maximize body language and posture, which supports the final pillar, that of appearance (Hewlett, 2016).

Appearance is grounded in dressing for the job that one wants, not the job one has. The institutional and professional leader's appearance should support one's ability to connect and communicate with others and represent one's unique brand or distinct appearance characteristic – the wearing of a broach, the wearing of a special type of bow tie, or the unique manner in which one presents oneself physically (Hewlett, 2016). Appearance should be commensurate with the context of the organizational culture and climate and appropriate to the given situation. Appearance communicates professionalism and respect for the executive position and others.

Growth Mindset

Our values, beliefs, paradigms, and perspectives influence our decisions and behaviors, and they formulate the mindset we use to interact with the world. One's mindset can be fixed or growth-oriented in nature. A *fixed mindset* has a perspective of static intelligence and is characterized by avoiding challenges, giving up on obstacles easily, perceiving effort as fruitless, avoiding negative or constructive criticism, and feeling threatened by the success of others. In contrast, a *growth mindset* has a perspective that intelligence can be developed and is characterized by embracing challenges, persisting in the face of obstacles, perceiving effort as the path to mastery, learning from criticism, and finding lessons and inspiration in the success of others (Dweck, 2016).

Effective academic leaders embrace a growth mindset which is based on a belief about cultivating the powerful passion for learning through stretching oneself and others to thrive during the most challenging times. From this perspective, failure is considered an opportunity, and effort is the key to success. With a growth mindset, effective leaders influence, motivate, and lead others in a "leadership space" outside of their comfort zone in an intentional and deliberate manner with the philosophy of improving and advancing all members of the community, achieving excellence rather than settling for mediocrity, and pursuing distinction for one's academic unit.

Emotional Intelligence

Relationships are considered the currency of leadership. A central concern in the discipline of nursing is "nursing civility." Leaders with emotional intelligence can manage their personal emotions and the ability to be in tune with other's emotional state without engaging in a negative reactionary manner. As respected nursing leaders, we are required to appropriately utilize our influence and power in a sometimes emotionally charged environment. Emotional intelligence provides the effective leader with earning power to gain relationship currency to advance their leadership ability.

Emotional intelligence is the ability to perceive the emotions of self and others, utilize emotions as a leadership tool, and understand the meaning of emotions to individuals, as well as maintain the regulation of emotions in light of a particular context (Goleman, 2005). There are four accepted components of emotional intelligence – self-awareness, self-management, social awareness, and relationship management. *Self-awareness* is the ability to recognize and understand personal emotions, moods, and drives, as well as their impact on others, and it has repeatedly been identified as an essential element of effective leadership. Self-awareness is considered the Hallmark characteristic of emotional intelligence since it consists of self-confidence, realistic self-assessment, and a self-deprecating sense of humor (Goleman, 2005).

Self-management is the ability to control or redirect disruptive impulses, moods, or emotions with the propensity of suspending judgment and thinking before acting. The essence of self-management is thinking before acting and avoiding the "amygdala hijacking" from our ingrained emotional responses. It consists, therefore, of self-control, transparency, adaptability, a drive for achievement, and initiative. *Social awareness* consists of empathy, organizational awareness, and service orientation, which allow an individual to appreciate the perspective of and empathize with others from diverse backgrounds, cultures, and social situations. *Relationship management* is built from the foundation of emotional awareness, self-management, and social awareness and is the ability to capitalize on one's interpersonal communication skills to motivate and inspire others through the bonds built with them. The essence of effective leadership is influencing and inspiring others to do something that they may not have done without that influence or inspiration. This is achieved through relationships – the currency of leadership. Relationship management consists of being inspirational, developing others, influencing others, acting as a change catalyst, managing conflict, building bonds, and engaging in teamwork and collaboration (Goleman, 2005).

FACULTY, ADMINISTRATORS, STUDENTS, AND ALUMNI PREPARE FOR AND ASSUME LEADERSHIP ROLES

The final Hallmark related to effective institutional and professional leadership is that faculty members, administrators, students, and alumni are prepared for and assume leadership roles that advance quality nursing care; promote positive change, innovation, and excellence; and enhance the impact of the nursing profession. The degree to which an academic unit has attained this Hallmark can be determined by the extent to which the following Indicators have been met: faculty members, administrators, and alumni serve on boards of partner institutions to improve quality and nursing care issues; faculty member, administrator, and student are recognized for the contributions of their work to the institution, profession, local community, or health care; the nursing curriculum and faculty development focus on leadership knowledge and skills; mentoring and development of future leaders is evident; members of the academic community are committed to creating and shaping a new reality for nursing education; and visionary dialogue about the future of nursing and nursing education occurs.

The ability of academic leaders to be prepared for and assume leadership roles within the academic, professional, local, national, and global communities is dependent upon their ability to prepare the next generation of leaders. As an effective leader this is our professional responsibility that can be achieved through framing and priming, engagement, mentoring, coaching, and succession planning.

Priming and Framing

To facilitate change and achieve excellence, effective institutional and professional leaders engage in policymaking and agenda setting that increases others' perception of the relevance of a new idea and the need to move it from merely an idea to an actionable item. Oftentimes, this is done by creating a sense of urgency, which is done through priming.

Priming is the placement of an issue within the mindset of others as a relevant and urgent area for change or policymaking. It is, in essence, a psychological process used to increase the salience of an issue through the activation of previously acquired information and to create a situational or institutional awareness through priming. In priming, an idea or concept about an issue or topic is planted within an individual's mind, and this "planting" facilitates the manner in which the individual thinks about or judges future information regarding that issue. It is through this priming mechanism that leaders influence "what others think about" as critical to the institutional or professional mission (Porche, 2018).

Framing complements the priming process by focusing attention on specific aspects of an issue while obscuring or decreasing the focus on other aspects of that issue; in essence, it provides the context and boundaries within which individuals think about an issue and the need for change. Leaders influence others by framing the paradigm from which to think about an issue which, in turn, helps align potential solutions with the leader's agenda (Porche, 2018).

Engagement

Engagement of members of any community is known to positively affect productivity, turnover, and profitability. In academe, engaged faculty members are more likely to remain within the academic institution and pursue leadership positions, and that engagement is dependent on the relationship with their academic leader. Academic environments that are characterized by strong relationships, feelings of inclusion, feeling needed by the institution and valued for one's unique skills and accomplishments, and opportunities to engage in activities that enhance one's personal and professional growth and development engage members of the community, promote advancement, and support efforts to achieve excellence and distinction (Pond, 2020). It is the academic leader who facilitates the development and ongoing support of such environments.

One framework academic leaders can use to promote such engagement is the engagement ring, where the **RING** represents **R**elationships, **I**nclusion, feeling **N**eeded, and **G**rowing. Relationships with the leader are critical to feeling encouraged and necessary for the building of a camaraderie that characterizes engagement. Engagement requires a sense of belonging and being included or kept "in the loop." Feeling needed is about having a sense of purpose and knowing that one's contributions to the institution or profession are important and valued; in other words, faculty or staff members who feel included and needed within an organization have a clear sense of how their personal and professional goals align with the institutional mission and vision, as well as how their "responsibilities and duties" actively contribute to the achievement of the academic mission. Lastly, Pond (2020) proposes growing is an element of engagement, and this growth can be promoted through "stretch" assignments that challenge faculty or staff and allow them to feel successful and be active contributors to the mission or goal. Pond (2020) espouses that the values of communication, constructive feedback, delegation, performance measurement, goals, and coaching are understood within the engagement ring.

Mentoring

Mentoring often is viewed as a factor that facilitates success. In fact, when we are asked to think about nursing colleagues who have achieved success and ask them how they achieved that success, many will say that one of the key factors that influenced and contributed to their success, regardless of their area of accomplishment, is the fact that they were mentored.

Mentoring is a reciprocal and collaborative relationship that can be formal or informal, but regardless of the type, its focus is on career development of the mentee. The two primary functions of a mentor are career-related or psychosocial. The *career-related function* establishes the mentor as an advisor who provides enhancement of the mentee's professional development and performance. The *psychosocial function* positions the mentor as a role model and support system for the mentee.

The mentoring relationship evolves through four stages – initiation, cultivation, separation, and redefinition. In the *initiation phase*, the mentor and mentee agree to and enter a mentoring relationship with each other; thus, true mentoring relationships are deliberate and explicit. During the *cultivation phase*, the work of mentoring occurs where both individuals focus on the goals and expectations of the relationship that generally include orientation, learning and professional development, and social network expansion. Successful *separation* is a phase that requires an open dialogue about the extent to which expectations of the mentoring relationship have been met, as well as open dialogue regarding the termination of the mentoring relationship. Many mentoring relationships are lifelong in which formal continual membership may have been terminated but there is a continual open relationship that provides for episodic mentoring to occur. Healthy mentoring relationships move from the separation phase of formal mentoring to a redefinition of the relationship. In the *redefinition stage*, the mentor and mentee relationship continues with a change in the focus and relationship dynamics that may (and often does) evolve into a mutual or peer type of mentoring relationship.

Mentoring relationships require a delineation of the roles and responsibilities of both the mentor and the mentee. Roles and responsibilities of the mentor typically include the following: relationship maintenance, sharing of self, honoring commitments to the mentee, maintaining confidentiality, being respectful and trustworthy, advising, educating, consulting, collaborating and guiding, coaching, helping to expand the mentee's networks, and serving as a resource person. Typical roles and responsibilities of the mentee include respecting the mentor's time and commitment, focusing on achieving learning goals, driving the mentoring relationship, creating SMART (specific, measurable, attainable, realistic and time bound) objectives, being authentic, being open and honest, preparing for meetings, taking responsibility to stay connected with the mentor, utilizing feedback, maintaining obligations, and engaging as a learner.

Mentoring is considered an effective leadership strategy for the promotion and development of future leaders and for helping individuals and groups achieve excellence and distinction. It can also be considered a professional obligation of all nurses.

Coaching

While mentors may engage in coaching, coaches are not necessarily mentors. The International Coaching Federation (ICF) provides the gold standard for what coaching really is. According to the ICF (2020), coaching is "partnering with clients in a thought-provoking and creative process that inspires them to maximize their personal and professional potential." In a coaching relationship, the coach is an accountability partner who utilizes powerful questioning as a strategy to elicit client-generated solutions. In other words, the coach does not provide solutions; instead, the client generates a personal action plan while the coach provides feedback on that plan and serves as a sounding board as the client implements it.

There are several coaching models that provide a framework for coaching relationships, one of which – the GOOD model – is simple and easy to use. It was developed by Auerbach (2001) and consists of four components – **G**oals, **O**pportunities, **O**bstacles, and **D**oing. *Goals* focus on the specific outcomes the client identified for a particular coaching session. It is the responsibility of the coach to remain flexible and fluid and continuously clarify the client's goals as the goals may change over the course of the relationship. In the coaching session, the coach queries the client on potential *opportunities* to achieve their goal. Through this process, the coach also challenges the client to identify potential *obstacles* or barriers to pursuing the stated opportunities to achieve their goal. The final aspect of the coaching model is *doing*, where the coach holds the client accountable for actionable behaviors.

Coaches utilize a variety of assessment tools to develop a deep understanding of the coaching client. These assessment tools permit the coach and client the opportunity to capitalize on the client as the strategic asset for change. Coaches serve as the accountability partner to ensure the leader emerges in effective leadership development.

Succession Planning

Succession planning is the formal process of identifying and developing future leaders who have the capability to assume a leadership position within an institution or organization in a timely manner. It utilizes mentoring and coaching as effective strategies to build the leadership pipeline and maximizes the availability of experienced and capable leaders with institutional knowledge and experience to assume leadership roles that become available.

In a spirit of effective institutional and professional leadership, succession planning is not a one-time activity; instead, it should be a continual strategy to ensure there is a constant pool of potential candidates for leadership roles. Therefore, succession planning requires a leadership paradigm that embraces valuing the ongoing development and engagement of members of the community – faculty, administrators, students, and alumni – so they are prepared to and do assume leadership roles. The succession planning process consists of the following activities that are nonlinear and iterative:

> Securing leadership support from upper level administrators

> Conducting an environmental scan of the profession

> Aligning succession planning with strategic initiatives and mission

> Assembling a succession planning team

> Determining management and leadership styles and competencies necessary for the respective organizational culture

> Examining leadership positions for vacancy risk and vacancy impact

> Reviewing existing leadership position descriptions for relevance and future leadership needs

> Identifying potential succession candidates

▸ Mapping leadership style and competency gaps between needed and desired leadership capability and potential succession candidates

▸ Initiating leadership development plans for succession candidates

▸ Continuing to improve the leadership succession planning process

CONCLUSION

It is clear that leaders carry the burden of the current moment, but they also carry the burden of planning for the future. Additionally, leaders are expected to meet society's demands for transparency, authenticity, and accountability.

Effective institutional and professional leaders are expected to be visionary, charismatic, mission focused, and strategic while developing a legacy and ensuring that the future is positive and optimistic. The NLN's Hallmarks that focus on leadership provide an opportunity for academic nursing leaders to leave a legacy of distinction while living their leadership journey of excellence. To be an authentic transformational leader, it is necessary to engage in a variety of leadership styles, remain emotionally intelligent, and be able to lead from all directions within an organization – lead in the front, lead as a follower, and lead laterally alongside other leaders. Strategies for developing distinctive excellence as a leader are summarized in Box 10-1, and when readers review and embrace these strategies, they are challenged to live, love, and enjoy their leadership journeys!

BOX 10-1

Effective Leadership Strategies for Creating Distinctive Excellence

- Communicate a clear vision, mission, and strategic direction.
- Be visible and accessible.
- Mentor everyone – formally and informally.
- Engage faculty, staff, and students into decision-making.
- Promote an open mindset.
- Support innovation and creativity.
- Create a sense of urgency for change.
- Capitalize on the power of positive moments.
- Exude executive presence.
- Maintain a growth mindset.
- Practice emotional intelligence.
- Focus on faculty, staff, and student engagement.
- Lead with character and authenticity.
- Collaborate across disciplines, within the academic institution, within the profession, and within the healthcare environment for strategic academic-practice partnerships.
- Promote a scholarly environment of inquiry.
- Create and promote a sense of institutional and professional citizenship.
- Promote integration of work and life balance into professional expectations for health and well-being.
- Role model and support professional association and community activities.
- Continually engage in environmental scanning for currency and relevance.

- Take responsibility, never place blame.
- Let go of power and control to be powerful.
- Listen more than you speak.
- Build solid teams with diverse personality profiles to generate creative and innovative solutions.
- Develop symbiotic relationships.
- Surround yourself with successful people.
- Know your core values.
- Build your leadership brand.
- Ensure that your reputation precedes you in a positive manner.
- Develop your resilience and grit.
- Promote rituals that support your desired culture and climate.
- Engage in the C's of leadership – cultivate, communicate, clarify, connect, collaborate, consult, coach, change, catalyze, create, cross-pollinate, and compassionate care.
- Engage in positive leadership with the expression of joy and happiness – never underestimate the healing power of laughter.

References

Ashby, F., & Pell, A. (2001). *Embracing excellence: Become an employer of choice to attract and keep the best talent.* Prentice Hall Press Publishers.

Auerbach, J. (2001). *Personal and executive coaching: Complete guide for mental health professionals.* Executive College Press.

Cavanaugh, A. (2016). *Contagious culture: Show up, set the tone, and intentionally create an organization that thrives.* McGraw-Hill Education.

Cavanaugh, A. (2020). *Contagious you: Unlock your power to influence, lead, and create the impact you want.* McGraw-Hill Education.

Coyle, D. (2018). *The culture code.* Bantam Books.

Dweck, C. (2016). *Mindset: The new psychology of success.* Penguin Random House LLC.

Gibson, R. (2015). *The four lenses of innovation: A power tool for creative thinking.* Wiley.

Goleman, D. (2005). *Emotional intelligence: Why it matters more than IQ.* Bantam Publishing.

Heath, C., & Health, D. (2017). *The power of moments.* Simon & Schuster.

Hewlett, S. (2016). *Executive presence: The missing link between merit and success.* HarperCollins Publishers.

International Coaching Federation. (2020). ICF definition of coaching. https://coachfederation.org/about

Kotter, J., & Cohen, D. (2002). *The heart of change: Real-life stories of how people change their organizations.* Harvard Business School Press.

National League for Nursing. (2020). *Hallmarks of excellence in nursing education model.* Author.

Pond, L. (2020). *The engagement ring: Practical leadership skills for engaging your employee.* Lioncrest Publishing.

Porche, D. (2018). *Health policy: Application for nurses and other health care professionals.* Jones & Bartlett Learning.

Schein, E. (2016). *Organizational culture and leadership* (5th ed.). Wiley.

11

Attaining Distinction in Nursing Education: National League for Nursing Programs Pave the Way

M. Elaine Tagliareni, EdD, RN, CNE, FAAN
Janice Brewington, PhD, RN, FAAN
Linda Christensen, EdD, JD, RN
Barbara Patterson, PhD, RN, FAAN, ANEF
Susan Gross Forneris, PhD, RN, CNE, CHSE-A, FAAN

INTRODUCTION

Throughout this book, authors have used the *Hallmarks of Excellence in Nursing Education*© (National League for Nursing [NLN], 2019) to boldly present ways nursing programs can pursue excellence to achieve distinction. The opening chapter clarifies that program approval by state boards and accreditation bodies are necessary and significant, but these designations do not necessarily set nursing programs apart, which is foundational to attaining distinction.

The NLN has a compelling and powerful history of championing excellence in nursing education. From its early days in 1893 through the 20th century, the Society of Superintendents of Training Schools for Nurses (the Society) and then the National League for Nursing Education (NLNE), led a movement to reform health care by bringing excellence and integrity to nursing education through development of curriculum guidelines, accreditation standards, and public policy reform initiatives (NLN, 2018). On the occasion of the NLN's centennial celebration in 1993, Dr. M. Louise Fitzpatrick spoke of this long-standing commitment to education, and in celebration of its 125th anniversary, the NLN reasserted its commitment to excellence by stating, "A mature profession with a more diverse and diffuse, but equally strong leadership, is our legacy. . . . It is our story and like the leaders of the past, we will continue to create it with distinction" (NLN, 2018, p. 9). This chapter provides an overview of the many NLN programs and initiatives that provide faculty and nursing programs with the opportunity to pursue excellence and attain distinction in nursing education, using the Hallmarks (NLN, 2019) as a guide.

HISTORY

Throughout the history of the NLN, the influence of the organization in accomplishing reform and the transformation of nursing and nursing education cannot be minimized. Since the inception of the organization, NLN leaders have developed a shared vision for the future of the nursing profession and clearly articulated strategies for advancing nursing education priorities.

During the 20th century, the Society, and then the NLNE, fully recognized the imperative to champion differences of ideas and perspectives while, at the same time, build models for standardization of national nursing curricula in the pursuit of reform and innovation. At the 1952 NLNE convention, when the NLNE joined with the National Organization of Public Health Nursing and the Association for Collegiate Schools of Nursing to become the NLN, Agnes Galina, president, called for nursing, and nurse educators in particular, to speak with one voice to establish "nursing education under the system of higher education of the country, providing qualified school personnel, and providing financial stability to the schools of nursing in America" (NLN, 2018, p. 64). From that time forward, the NLN has consistently pursued policies and programming for nurse educators to employ quality teaching practices, build curricula that are informed by practice and sound principles, and create a culture that reflects a commitment to pedagogical scholarship and continuous quality improvement. The current Hallmarks (NLN, 2019) build on that legacy and provide guidance for achieving excellence and distinction in nursing education so that graduates are prepared to be successful in and have a positive impact on today's complex healthcare environment.

As the 20th century was nearing its end, NLN leaders recognized the need to provide programming that would assist faculty, and nursing programs, to move beyond traditional ways of demonstrating excellence and achieve distinction. With that intent, a flurry of activity occurred at the NLN, and new programming to illustrate notable achievements by faculty and nursing programs emerged.

The NLN Board of Governors expressed interest in and support of a "Magnet school" concept and encouraged thinking about how the NLN could promote excellence in all types of academic programs and offer schools/colleges of nursing the opportunity to receive an externally awarded designation that recognizes their innovative and distinctive efforts in selected areas. In 2004, the NLN awarded the Centers of Excellence in Nursing Education™ (COE) designation for the first time to schools/colleges of nursing that had achieved a level of sustained, evidence-based, and substantive innovation in advancing the science of nursing education and enhancing student learning and professional development. By 2011, the NLN expanded the COE program to healthcare organizations, recognizing that these institutions play a significant role in promoting the academic progression of nurses.

One year before COE designations were first awarded, the NLN established the Certified Nurse Educator (CNE®) program to give national recognition to nursing education as a specialty area of practice and provide a means for faculty to demonstrate their expertise in this role. By 2005, a practice analysis was completed and the psychometrically sound inaugural CNE examination was piloted, launching a national movement to validate the expertise of nurse educators.

Acknowledging that certification was a mark of expertise as an educator, the NLN then moved to establish a way to recognize the leadership provided by nurse educators and the impact of their substantial contributions to the field. The answer to this quest was to establish the Academy of Nursing Education, and in 2007 the inaugural group of the Academy of Nursing Education Fellows (ANEF) was inducted. The enduring and substantial contributions to nursing education made by these and subsequent Fellows have been through their roles as teachers, mentors, scholars, public policy advocates, practice partners, and administrators.

In 2007 the NLN Board of Governors recognized the imperative to revise the NLN mission, goals, and core values to more fully reflect the NLN's mission to promote excellence in nursing education, to champion nurse educators in the pursuit of excellence, and to create pathways to acknowledge that excellence. The mission clearly reflects the NLN's core values – caring, integrity, diversity, and excellence – that are foundational to all NLN initiatives. This clear sense of purpose led to the formulation of goals to (1) continue NLN's legacy of leadership in nursing education, (2) define its strong and sustained commitment to members, (3) champion nurse educators by expanding opportunities for their professional advancement and recognizing theirs as an advanced practice role, and (4) promote research and scholarship that advances the science of nursing education.

In the next decade, the NLN expanded its mission statement to embrace the original mission of the Superintendents' Society, to unite nursing education and practice in pursuit of safe patient care, to "advance the health of the nation," and to include the global community. That mission is shown in Box 11-1.

Considering its renewed commitment to the global community as well as the national one, the NLN partnered with CGFNS International to expand its CNE program so that educators from around the globe are eligible to sit for the certification exam. And in recognition of the critical but more focused scope of practice of those who teach primarily in clinical settings, the organization introduced the Certified Academic Clinical Nurse Educator (CNEcl) program as a means of validating expertise in that specific role.

In 2012, the NLN introduced its now signature Leadership Institute to provide learning opportunities for nurse leaders across all career trajectories, from aspiring/emerging to experienced, to maximize their leadership potential and make a difference in their home institutions and in the broader educational community. The organization has enhanced its commitment to advancing the science of nursing education through publication of priorities for research in nursing education, expansion of its research and dissertation grants program, and increasing the capacity of the NLN's peer-reviewed

BOX 11-1

Mission of the National League for Nursing 2019–2021

The National League for Nursing promotes excellence in nursing education to build a strong and diverse nursing workforce to advance the health of our nation and the global community.

journal, *Nursing Education Perspectives*, through its strategic partnership with Wolters Kluwer. Additionally, the NLN increased its focus on publications, online resources, workshops, and other scholarly activities to provide opportunities for nurse educators to disseminate their scholarly work and enhance their pedagogical knowledge. All these initiatives promote excellence in nursing education and provide opportunities for schools to achieve distinction.

This whirlwind of activity clearly exemplifies the NLN's mission-driven dedication to support nurse educators and nursing programs in their pursuit of excellence and in their determination to attain distinction in nursing education. Several of the key initiatives designed to promote excellence and acknowledge individuals and schools that have achieved distinction are described further in the subsequent pages.

CENTERS OF EXCELLENCE (COE) PROGRAM

The NLN's commitment to excellence in nursing education, its work to encourage schools to strive toward excellence, and its strategic goal to create a program that provides support to institutions to achieve that goal is at the core of the COE program (NLN, n.d. e). The COE program criteria are designed to recognize the unique strengths of a school/college of nursing relative to the NLN mission, and to set high standards that distinguish and publicly recognize those schools in one of the following areas: (1) creating environments that promote the pedagogical expertise of faculty; (2) creating environments that enhance student learning and professional development; (3) creating environments that advance the science of nursing education; and (4) creating workplace environments that promote the academic progression of nurses.

Background

At the turn of this century, the NLN took bold steps to reorganize its structure, uniting its membership as one faculty dedicated to engaging in dialogue to transform nursing education and practice. Several committees were formed to execute this goal. The Nursing Education Advisory Council (NEAC) was formed to provide leadership in curriculum design, promote strategies that facilitate the continuous quality improvement of all nursing programs, encourage innovation, and advance best practices in nursing education. One of NEAC's first endeavors was to develop the COE program. Members of NEAC identified that nursing programs were looking to distinguish themselves from one another as a way of attracting and retaining outstanding faculty and exceptional students; they also noted that although the ANCC Magnet program was gaining national prominence in hospitals across the nation, schools/colleges of nursing had few opportunities to receive an externally awarded designation that recognized their innovative and excellent efforts in specific areas.

With full endorsement from the NLN Board of Governors, NLN members who served on NEAC developed the criteria and structure of the COE program to distinguish those schools that demonstrate evidence-based, substantive innovation in a selected area; conduct ongoing research to document the effectiveness of such innovation; set high standards for themselves; and commit to continuous improvement. Such recognition would indicate a commitment by the school/college to pursue and sustain excellence in student learning and professional development, ongoing faculty development, or nursing education research.

Impact of the Center of Excellence Program

The criteria for COE designation clearly align with the Hallmarks (NLN, 2019). For example, criteria in the COE category of *Creating Environments that Enhance Student Learning and Professional Development* align with Hallmarks related directly to engaged students; innovative, evidence-based curriculum; innovative, evidence-based approaches to facilitate and evaluate learning; and commitment to pedagogical scholarship. Criteria in the COE category of *Creating Environments that Promote the Pedagogical Expertise of Faculty* relate clearly to Hallmarks that address a diverse, well-prepared faculty; a culture of continuous quality improvement; resources to support program goal attainment; and effective institutional and professional leadership. And Hallmarks that address a diverse, well-prepared faculty; innovative, evidence-based curriculum; innovative, evidence-based approaches to facilitate and evaluate learning; and commitment to pedagogical scholarship align clearly with the COE category of *Creating Environments that Advance the Science of Nursing Education*. Faculty, therefore, can use the Hallmarks – perhaps through the self-assessment tool included as Appendix C – to determine their readiness to apply for COE designation.

Over the course of the past two decades, schools/colleges that have achieved COE designation have identified benefits of being nationally recognized for excellence. These nursing programs are proud that their work, to impact the health of the nation by building a strong and diverse nursing workforce, has been recognized and rewarded. Applying for this recognition has encouraged discussions among faculty, students, program graduates, and employers about excellence in nursing education and how the school/college of nursing operationalizes excellence. Additionally, nursing schools/colleges with this designation have taken the lead in facilitating positive changes that re-form nursing education based on the application of evidence gleaned from research in practice and education, as well as the development of innovative education-practice partnerships. Designation as an NLN Center of Excellence in Nursing Education is an accomplishment that sets a school/college apart from other schools/colleges, highlights its unique strengths, serves as a strong factor in marketing it to prospective students and faculty, encourages enhanced alumni engagement and strong partnerships with key stakeholders, and honors the school both within and outside its own institution. These distinctive programs exemplify and role model visionary leadership, substantive innovation, and environments of inclusive excellence.

ACADEMIC NURSE EDUCATOR CERTIFICATION PROGRAMS

The NLN's mission to be a champion for nurse educators and to advocate for equity and recognition in the advanced practice role of nurse educator is actualized in the development and implementation of the Academic Nurse Educator Certification Programs (NLN, n.d. b). There are currently two NLN nurse educator certifications. The CNE program, introduced in 2005, is a means of validating an individual's expertise in the full scope of the role of academic nurse educator. The CNEcl program, launched in 2018, is a means of validating an individual's expertise in the specific role of academic clinical nurse educator. As of mid-2020, approximately 8,000 academic nurse educators have attained the credential of CNE, and approximately 300 academic clinical nurse educators have attained the credential of CNEcl.

Background

As of the early 2000s, there was no evidence-based or research-based description of the academic nurse educator role. Most nursing faculty entered the role of educator without any formal preparation for it, and they often approached teaching as they were taught, as mentored by senior colleagues, or by trial and error. The NLN actively promoted the role of the academic nurse educator by promoting lifelong learning for nursing faculty to remain current in the role as an educator (NLN, 2001), identifying the role as one requiring specialized preparation, and publishing a position that teaching nursing is an advanced practice role that requires specialized knowledge and skills (NLN, 2005). In response to the lack of a clearly defined nurse educator role, the NLN created a Task Group on Nurse Educator Competencies. Between 2002 and 2004, the Task Group completed an extensive review of the literature resulting in the development of the NLN Core Competencies of Nurse Educators© and publication of a book (Halstead, 2007) that explicated the competencies and provided the evidence on which each was based. The eight core competencies reflected the full scope of the role of the academic nurse educator and provided the initial framework for the creation of the CNE program.

As academic nursing programs struggled to find sufficient numbers of qualified nurse educators to fill full-time positions and hired more individuals to focus primarily or solely on teaching in the clinical or laboratory setting, the NLN convened a task group in 2007 to complete an extensive review of the literature regarding clinical nursing education in order to identify the core competencies for this role. The resulting six core competencies were validated through a practice analysis and eventually provided the initial framework for the creation of the Academic Clinical Nurse Educator certification program.

Impact of Nurse Educator Certification

The attainment of certification in nursing signifies proficiency in a specific set of competencies associated with a role or specialty. For the individual academic nurse educator, the designation of CNE or CNEcl indicates that the individual has demonstrated competence in either the full scope of the academic nurse educator role or the more limited-in-scope academic clinical nurse educator role. The individual CNE or CNEcl is distinguished by the ability to put the credential "CNE" or "CNEcl" after their name. The NLN certification has earned national and international acknowledgement of meeting the professional competencies associated with the professional nurse educator role. Although nurse educator certification is voluntary, earning the credential is associated with professional recognition and self-satisfaction for the individual.

Both of NLN's certification programs are grounded in evidence-based competencies, and the CNE competencies are closely aligned with the NLN Hallmarks (NLN, 2019). For example, the CNE competencies of using assessment and evaluation strategies and participation in curriculum design and evaluation of programs align with Hallmarks in the categories of continuous quality improvement and innovative, evidence-based curricula, as well as evidence-based strategies to facilitate and evaluate learning. The CNE competency of engaging in scholarship, service, and leadership is closely associated with Hallmarks of commitment to pedagogical scholarship and effective institutional and professional leadership.

In addition to affirming the scope of responsibilities of academic nurse educators and academic clinical nurse educators, CNE competencies have been used as a framework for the development of graduate programs designed to prepare nurse educators (Fitzgerald et al., 2020). The CNE competencies also have been included within faculty position descriptions, faculty development programs, and faculty evaluations. As the CNEcl competencies are still considered relatively new, they have not yet been used as extensively as the CNE competencies; however, anecdotal reports to the NLN (L. Simmons, personal communication, September 1, 2020) indicate that the CNEcl competencies provide a comprehensive framework for being used in the creation of clinical nurse educator orientation programs.

FELLOWSHIP IN THE ACADEMY OF NURSING EDUCATION

The NLN's mission to champion nurse educators by building equity and recognition in the advanced practice role of nurse educators reached another milestone in 2007 when the NLN launched the Academy of Nursing Education program to recognize faculty and others who have made an enduring and substantial contribution to the field of nursing education. Establishing the Academy was an historic step for the NLN, and it provided a way for nurse educators to be distinguished as leaders whose wisdom and scholarship advanced nursing education. To be awarded the distinction of being an NLN Fellow, entitled to use the approved credential of ANEF (Academy of Nursing Education Fellow), provided long overdue stature to the nurse educator role.

Background

In 2005, members of the NEAC, in collaboration with the NLN Board of Governors, conceived the idea of initiating a recognition program for nurse educators. Members of the NEAC identified that recognizing nurse educators would create distinction for the role; additionally, development of an Academy that acknowledged the sustained and significant contributions of nursing educator leaders would foster excellence by capitalizing on the wisdom of outstanding individuals inside and outside the profession. These individuals would provide visionary leadership for nursing programs, for the NLN, and for the national and global nursing education enterprise, in full support of the mission and core values of the NLN.

Criteria focusing on the individual's contributions to nursing education in teaching/learning innovations, faculty development, research in nursing education, leadership in nursing education, public policy related to nursing education, and/or collaborative education/practice/community partnerships were established. Potential candidates would be required to be current members of the NLN, whether individually or through their schools, and be asked to show how they already have and would continue to provide leadership in the development of pedagogical scholarship and research and in the preparation of a nursing workforce that meets the needs of an ever-changing healthcare environment. At the 2007 NLN Education Summit, the inaugural class of 41 Fellows, representing 33 schools of nursing throughout the nation, was inducted. Since then, more than 300 nurse educators have been accepted into the Academy; these leading nurse educators teach in a range of programs across the spectrum of higher education and are affiliated with exemplary teaching hospitals and other organizations committed to advancing excellence in nursing education and quality health care in the United States and globally.

Impact of the Academy

The NLN Academy of Nursing Education (NLN, n.d. a) has, over the past 13 years, established a track record of significant contributions to nursing education, the nursing profession, and the NLN. Academy Fellows were involved in updating and refining the Hallmarks (NLN, 2019) by providing input to revisions of categories and Indicators, as well as by serving as expert advisors for relevance and applicability of the Hallmarks. Academy Fellows embrace the full scope of the academic nurse educator role, specifically exemplifying the Hallmarks of innovative and evidence-based curriculum, innovative and evidence-based approaches to facilitate and evaluate learning, commitment to pedagogical scholarship, and effective institutional and professional leadership.

Fellows in the NLN's Academy of Nursing Education serve as important role models to novice and mid-career nurse educators, assisting them to aspire to make a difference in nursing education, which ultimately impacts the health of the nation and global community. They serve as mentors and resources, both nationally and globally, to champion the role and to advocate for the validity and importance of excellence in teaching nursing. As noted by NLN President Patricia Yoder-Wise on the occasion of the announcement of the 2020 Fellows, Academy members play a "critical role in preparing nursing school graduates to step right onto the front lines to deliver sustainable, accessible, culturally-sensitive care to a diverse patient population and demonstrate anew why nurses are considered the most trusted professionals in health care today" (NLN, 2020a). The distinction of being an ANEF is the highest honor in nursing education leadership bestowed by the NLN as it salutes teachers, mentors, scholars, public policy advocates, practice partners, and administrators who have made an enduring and substantial contribution to the field of nursing education.

LEADERSHIP DEVELOPMENT PROGRAMS

In light of the increasing complexity of academic institutions, health systems, and the external environment, nurses must be positioned to provide leadership within all types of organizations. Achieving excellence and distinction are not easily awarded – they must be achieved through purposeful development of knowledge and skill. Nursing education leaders, both formal and informal, transform schools of nursing through initiatives that support effective student engagement, outstanding teaching, and a vibrant community of educators and learners who are committed to achieving targeted outcomes with distinction. Recognizing this reality, the NLN Center for Transformational Leadership Institute, in collaboration with the NLN Center for Innovation in Education Excellence, currently offers two leadership development programs: LEAD and the Leadership Development Program for Simulation Educators (NLN, n.d. c). The goal of both programs is to ensure that faculty constituents have access to resources and programs that promote excellence and use foundational leadership principles. Graduates of the programs use the knowledge, skills, and insights gained from their experiences to shape a preferred future for nursing education.

Background

When the Institute of Medicine (IOM) released *The Future of Nursing: Leading Change, Advancing Health* (IOM, 2011) and made recommendations for an action-oriented blueprint for the future of nursing, the NLN moved swiftly to address the report's recommendation to prepare and enable nurses to lead change to advance health. The simulation leader program began that year with a goal to maximize the leadership potential of experienced simulation nurse educators to advance simulation initiatives in nursing education and practice. This program was followed in 2011 with another one-year intensive program, LEAD, a program designed for individuals transitioning into leadership positions, individuals in administrative positions who had never engaged in a formal leadership development program, and individuals aspiring to lead in the future. Each program has its own distinctive focus and objectives, and each engages its participants in collaborative learning to co-create strategies to enhance their leadership skills and their ability to engage in change management and transformative planning for their organizations. Participants are challenged to use the authority inherent in their formal positions, as well as their personal authority, to influence innovation for their organization's future. These programs are in direct alignment with the NLN Hallmarks (NLN, 2019) that address effective institutional and professional leadership, which calls for leaders to be prepared for and assume leadership roles that advance quality nursing care; promote positive change, innovation, and excellence; and enhance the impact of the nursing profession.

Impact of Leadership Programs

Distinction is achieved using an intentional process of faculty engagement to develop excellence and leadership skills. The implications can be seen in three main themes of outcomes shared by NLN faculty members who have been involved in NLN's leadership programs.

Access to Formal Leaders

The two leadership programs offered by the NLN utilize elements of shared leadership with cohorts of faculty leaders working together and engaging in powerful dialogue to share wisdom and perspectives on – and propose solutions to – significant challenges in nursing education. The opportunity to connect with colleagues and obtain perspectives outside one's own community creates a dynamic collaboration. Leaders *lead each other* in a shared community. This shared journey expands professional networks and enhances the capacity of participants to adapt strategies and qualities of others to develop their own authentic leadership style for success in achieving organizational outcomes.

Interpersonal Development Through Leadership Innovation

Highly accomplished role models assist participants to see both formal and informal leadership in action and provide multiple opportunities for participants to reflect carefully on their beliefs, enhance their interpersonal skills, and envision the contributions they hope to make to the discipline. Excellence and distinction are formed as both formal and informal leaders collaborate to achieve skills in the areas of communication competence, conflict management, positive influence, successful team building, and encouragement of innovative thinking. Pathways for ongoing interpersonal development emerge.

Improving Education Outcomes

Those who have participated in the NLN leadership programs have voiced a new clarity and understanding related to the significance of and their contributions to the larger organizational picture, the importance of culture, the effective use of power, and the ways in which these concepts interrelate to one another. Ultimately, their roles as leaders impact their organizations' mission, they develop a new sense of empowerment, and they understand and operationalize their roles to drive the organizations' success. Their distinction as emerging leaders and their new voice have a positive influence on the way the organization moves and achieves outcomes.

The inclusive outcome for participants is leadership excellence, which is consistently integrated in their leadership roles. Leadership excellence serves as the foundation for organizations to build capacity and sustainability and provides participants the opportunity to attain distinction within their organizations.

SCHOLARSHIP DEVELOPMENT INITIATIVES

Through multiple initiatives, the NLN has supported the generation, translation, and dissemination of robust scholarship related to nursing education. These initiatives include the creation of research priorities in nursing education (NLN, 2020b), the nursing education research and dissertation grants program (NLN, n.d. d), the Scholarly Writing Retreat (NLN, n.d. f), and scholarly dissemination through books, journal articles, and presentations at conferences. They are aligned with the spirit of inquiry promoted by the NLN and provide opportunities to influence the future of nursing education.

Background

Advancing the science of nursing education has been a priority for the NLN for more than three decades, and it serves to distinguish the organization from others. Recognizing the need for rigorous scholarship in nursing education, the NLN established research priorities, provided funding to support research and other scholarly activities, and supported efforts to disseminate evidence that enhance faculty teaching practice.

Engaging in scholarship is a core competency for the nurse educator (Halstead, 2019), the COE category that focuses on advancing the science of nursing education and the NLN Hallmarks (NLN, 2019) that address a commitment to pedagogical scholarship. Indicators for that Hallmark challenge faculty to reflect on ways in which they and students promote scholarly inquiry related to nursing education, as well as the strategies used to systematically document the extent to which student learning experiences affect healthcare outcomes for the populations they serve.

Scholarship is a moral imperative and the "responsibility of all academic nurse educators as disciplinary stewards to prepare the future nursing workforce and promote optimal health care outcomes locally, nationally, and globally" (Patterson & McLaughlin, 2019, p. 135). The NLN's distinction to support nurse faculty and colleges/schools of nursing in the development of scholarship has been significant and long-standing.

Priorities for Research in Nursing Education

Every three years the NLN updates the research priorities for nursing education (NLN, 2020b) based on emergent and future-oriented foci relevant to nursing education and faculty teaching practice. As the science of nursing education and learning science evolve and grow, areas that require greater evidence must be examined, and these priorities provide direction and support for investigators as they design their research. Closely linked with the NLN grants program, investigators must also demonstrate linkage of their research to the priorities.

Nursing Education Research and Dissertation Grants Program

Over the past 20 years, the NLN nursing education research grants program (NLN, n.d. d) has funded more than 120 individual research projects, distributing approximately 1.25 million in research grant dollars. Currently, principal investigators can request up to $30,000 for a 1- to 2-year research project. Additionally, through several co-sponsored awards, doctoral students can submit grant requests to support their dissertation research. The diversity of funded topics is broad, from instrument development to experimental designs and qualitative studies that focus on understanding educational experiences from the perspective of both students and faculty. Investigators are encouraged to design global and multisite studies to extend the impact of the generated evidence.

Scholarly Dissemination

The NLN Scholarly Writing Retreat (NLN, n.d. f) is a year-long mentored program to help faculty enhance their writing skills and publish their work. This initiative has been offered twice a year for more than a decade, and in the past five years more than 130 faculty have participated. With the goal of submitting a manuscript to a scholarly journal at the conclusion of the retreat, the impact of this program has been outstanding with approximately 90 percent of faculty achieving publication within a year and multiple participants publishing two manuscripts in that time period.

In partnership with Wolters Kluwer Publishing, the NLN has been at the forefront of publishing books and a journal relevant to nursing faculty scholarship and teaching practice grounded in empirical evidence and pedagogical theory. For example, a recent publication, *Critical Conversations (Vol. 2): Moving from Monologue to Dialogue* (Forneris & Fey, 2020), offers guidance and new teaching approaches for faculty to engage students based on evidence from learning science. The NLN journal, *Nursing Education Perspectives*, is a leading source for current research and innovative ideas focused on academic nursing education. Published six times per year and an NLN member benefit, the journal editors strive to publish cutting edge research critical to providing faculty with a foundation for evidence-based teaching practice.

Scholarship in nursing academia is foundational for the development of the science of nursing education. Nursing academia values scholarship, and the NLN's initiatives demonstrate its commitment to scholarship. Faculty need robust evidence to inform their teaching practice to prepare the next generation of nurses, advanced practice nurses, nurse educators, and leaders to be at the forefront of the discipline. These initiatives position institutions to be able to achieve their goals, be recognized as excellent, and support the development of faculty as nurse scholars, scientists, and leaders, as well as teachers who implement best teaching practices.

CONCLUSION

Faculty in schools of nursing are responding to the call for excellence in their work as nurse educators. Excellence in nursing education has multiple components as presented in this book. This chapter has provided an overview of NLN programs that provide faculty and nursing programs the opportunity to pursue excellence and attain distinction in nursing education, using the Hallmarks (NLN, 2019) as benchmarks to achieve this goal. NLN programs that recognize nurse educators and nursing programs for leadership and demonstrate competency in the nurse educator role, institutional quality, and faculty scholarship align with the NLN's mission to promote excellence in nursing education and to lead in setting standards that advance excellence and innovation in nursing education. As a dedicated champion for nurse educators, the NLN will continue its powerful historical legacy to bring excellence, distinction, transformative reform, and innovation to nursing education and to the work of the NLN.

References

Fitzgerald, A., McNelis, A. M., & Billings, D. M. (2020). NLN core competencies for nurse educators: Are they present in the course descriptions of academic nurse educator programs? *Nursing Education Perspectives*, 41(1), 4–12. https:doi.org///10.1097/01 .NEP.0000000000000530

Forneris, S. G., & Fey, M. K. (2020). *Critical conversations (Vol. 2): Moving from monologue to dialogue*. National League for Nursing.

Halstead, J. A. (Ed.). (2007). *Nurse educator competencies: Creating an evidence-based practice for nurse educators*. National League for Nursing.

Halstead, J. A. (Ed.). (2019). *NLN core competencies for nurse educators: A decade of influence*. National League for Nursing.

Institute of Medicine. (2011). *The future of nursing: Leading change, advancing health*. National Academies Press.

National League for Nursing. (2001). *Position statement: Lifelong learning for nursing faculty*. http://www.nln.org/docs/default-source/about/archived-position-statements/lifelong-learning-for-nursing-faculty-pdf.pdf?sfvrsn=8

National League for Nursing. (2005). *Transforming nursing education*. http://www.nln.org/docs/default-source/about/archived-position-statements/transforming052005.pdf?sfvrsn=6

National League for Nursing. (2018). *Celebrating 125 years of leadership in nursing education; Inspiring words: Selected NLN addresses 1893–present*. http://www.nln.org/docs/default-source/about/commemorativebook2018-11-single-page.pdf?sfvrsn=2

National League for Nursing. (2019). *Hallmarks of excellence in nursing education*. http://www.nln.org/professional-development-programs/teaching-resources/hallmarks-of-excellence

National League for Nursing. (2020a). *News release: NLN welcomes new fellows' class into the Academy of Nursing Education*. http://www.nln.org/newsroom/news-releases/news-release/2020/08/07/nln-welcomes-new-fellows-class-into-the-academy-of-nursing-education

National League for Nursing. (2020b). *NLN research priorities in nursing education 2020–2023*. http://www.nln.org/docs/default-source/Research-Grants/nln-research-priorities-in-nursing-education.pdf?sfvrsn=0

National League for Nursing. (n.d. a). *Academy of nursing education*. http://www.nln.org/recognition-programs/academy-of-nursing-education

National League for Nursing. (n.d. b). *Certification for nurse educators*. http://www.nln.org/Certification-for-Nurse-Educators

National League for Nursing. (n.d. c). *NLN leadership institute*. http://www.nln.org/professional-development-programs/leadership-programs

National League for Nursing. (n.d. d). *NLN nursing education research grants program*. http://www.nln.org/professional-development-programs/grants-and-scholarships/nursing-education-research-grants

National League for Nursing. (n.d. e). *Purpose and goals of the COE program*. http://www.nln.org/recognition-programs/centers-of-excellence-in-nursing-education/purpose- and-goals-of-the-coe-program

National League for Nursing. (n.d. f). *Scholarly writing retreat: An NLN mentoring program*. http://www.nln.org/centers-for-nursing-education/nln-chamberlain-university-college-of-nursing-center-for-the-advancement-of-the-science-of-nursing-education2/scholarly-writing-retreat

Patterson, B., & McLaughlin, K. (2019). Competency VII: Engage in scholarship. In J. A. Halstead (Ed.), *NLN core competencies for nurse educators: A decade of influence* (pp. 135–148). National League for Nursing.

Appendix A
Hallmarks of Excellence in Nursing Education Model

HALLMARKS OF EXCELLENCE IN NURSING EDUCATION MODEL

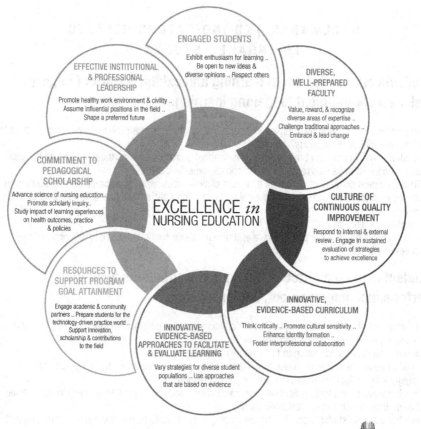

Copyright © April 2020. National League for Nursing

Note: The *Hallmarks of Excellence in Nursing Education Model©*, along with the individual components of it in various chapters of this book, are included with the permission of the National League for Nursing.

Appendix B
Hallmarks of Excellence in Nursing Education with Indicators

Note: The *Hallmarks of Excellence in Nursing Education©* and Indicators are included here with the permission of the National League for Nursing.

HALLMARKS AND INDICATORS RELATED TO ENGAGED STUDENTS

Students are excited about learning and exhibit a spirit of inquiry as well as a commitment to lifelong learning.

- To what extent do students appraise evidence and use the information discovered to contribute to class and clinical discussions?
- In what ways do students brainstorm together about concepts such as those presented in class and introduced in various references and clinical experiences?
- To what extent do students question if current clinical practices (e.g., approaches to patient care, the way communication occurs on clinical units, existing policies) are based on research and evidence?
- Do students ask "What if" questions?
- In what ways do students demonstrate enthusiasm about continued learning and professional development?

Students are committed to innovation, continuous quality/performance improvement, and excellence.

- To what extent do students respond to critical/constructive feedback and then use that feedback to make improvements in their performance?
- In what ways are students open to trying new things?
- In what ways are students stimulated in their learning when innovative teaching strategies are integrated into the classroom, lab, and/or clinical setting?
- In what ways do students reflect on their own performance and experiences in order to be proactive in implementing improved performance?
- In what ways do students observe for areas of quality improvement within systems and suggest appropriate solutions?
- In what ways are students incorporating technology to make improvements in their performance?

Students are committed to the professional nursing role including advancement in leadership, scholarship, and mentoring.

- In what ways do students express anticipatory excitement about professional identity formation, continuing their education, pursuing graduate study, assuming leadership roles in their employment settings and in the profession, serving as mentors, and becoming actively involved in professional associations? How do they express excitement about the contributions they hope to make to the nursing profession?
- In what ways do students propose a realistic short- and long-term career trajectory for themselves?
- To what extent do students collaborate with others to create environments that are civil, inclusive, respectful, and promote excellence?
- In what ways do students provide evidence of seeing themselves as being responsible for advancing the profession of nursing?

HALLMARKS AND INDICATORS RELATED TO DIVERSE, WELL-PREPARED FACULTY

The faculty complement is composed of diverse individuals who are leaders and/or have expertise in clinical practice, education, interprofessional collaboration, and research/scholarship consistent with the parent institution's mission and vision.

- To what extent does the faculty complement reflect diversity, including but not limited to race, ethnicity, gender, and educational background?
- To what extent do hiring practices help to create a faculty complement that reflects expertise in education, clinical practice, interprofessional collaboration, and/or research/scholarship?
- To what extent do faculty members' job responsibility statements specifically address the expert behaviors required for the roles of educator, clinician, and researcher/scholar?

The unique contributions of each faculty member in teaching, service, research/scholarship, and practice that facilitate achievement of the program's mission and goals are valued, rewarded, and recognized.

- To what extent are the unique contributions of faculty members with varied areas of expertise valued, rewarded, and recognized?
  - Expertise in education
  - Expertise in clinical practice
  - Expertise in research/scholarship
  - Expertise in interprofessional collaboration
  - Expertise in administration and/or management

Faculty members are accountable for promoting excellence, creating civil and inclusive environments, and providing leadership in their area(s) of expertise.

- How are faculty members expected to demonstrate expertise and promote diversity?
- How do expert faculty members provide leadership and mentoring to other faculty members regarding their area(s) of expertise?
- In what ways are faculty members held accountable to fulfill expectations related to diversity, excellence, and providing leadership in their area(s) of expertise?
- In what ways do faculty members actively work to promote academic integrity and sustain an environment of civility and inclusivity?
- To what extent have faculty members made a commitment to challenge traditional approaches to nursing education and implement innovative, evidence-based approaches?

Faculty members model a commitment to lifelong learning, involvement in professional and community organizations, and scholarly activities.

- To what extent do faculty members demonstrate an openness to embracing and leading change in the learning environment and acquiring needed faculty competencies to create a preferred future in nursing?
- To what extent are faculty members expected to continue learning and acquiring knowledge in their area(s) of expertise through continuing education courses, certifications, post-master's courses, post-doctoral courses, or other formal or informal education?
- To what extent do faculty members make significant contributions to local, state, regional, national, and/or international professional organizations?
- To what extent do faculty members express excitement about a professional career in nursing when talking with students, with one another, and with others inside and outside the profession?

All faculty members have structured preparation for the faculty role, including competence in teaching, scholarship, and service.

- Do all full-time, part-time, and adjunct faculty members receive an in-depth orientation to the faculty role?
- What forms of mentorship are provided to assist faculty members as they progress in their careers?
- Is an established set of faculty competencies used to prepare individuals for the faculty role and help them maintain competence or expertise in that role?

HALLMARKS AND INDICATORS RELATED TO A CULTURE OF CONTINUOUS QUALITY IMPROVEMENT

The program engages in a variety of activities that promote quality and excellence, including accreditation by national nursing accreditation bodies.

- In what ways does the school's strategic plan reflect findings from the continuous quality improvement process in which faculty members, students, administrators, alumni, and community partners participate?
- To what extent does the program have a process to support faculty research/scholarship; attendance at local, national, and international conferences; and faculty development events?
- Does each program seek and maintain national nursing accreditation?
- To what extent are accreditation standards used to guide program evaluation and develop a culture of continuous quality improvement of the nursing program?

Program design, implementation, and evaluation are continuously reviewed and revised to achieve and maintain excellence.

- Is there a mechanism in place for continuous review of program design, implementation, and evaluation?
- In what ways are curricular revisions made that allow the program to keep current with changes and trends in health care, healthcare economics, healthcare delivery systems, education, national standards and competencies, societal norms, and expectations of nurses?
- In what ways are faculty members, along with administrators, engaged in discussion about quality improvement as part of their role within the organization?
- To what extent are program revisions based on findings from the continuous review of program design, implementation, and evaluation?
- To what extent do faculty members and students systematically evaluate the impact of innovative teaching strategies and curriculum approaches on (1) student learning outcomes, student satisfaction, and other student-centered outcomes; and (2) faculty satisfaction, scholarship, and professional growth?

HALLMARKS AND INDICATORS RELATED TO INNOVATIVE, EVIDENCE-BASED CURRICULUM

The curriculum is designed to help students achieve stated program outcomes, reflects current societal and healthcare trends and issues, and is responsive to change and evolving societal needs. The curriculum also embeds evidence-based information, reflects research findings and innovative practices, attends to the evolving role of the nurse in a variety of settings, is flexible and innovative, and incorporates local, national, and global perspectives.

- What opportunities are available for students to take courses in a sequence that makes sense to them or allows them to pursue study in areas in which they have learning needs?
- To what extent is the curriculum offered in flexible formats (e.g., part-time/full-time, day/evening, online/face-to-face/hybrid) to meet the individualized needs of students?
- To what extent is the curriculum flexible, allowing faculty members to address new issues, new knowledge and scientific developments, emerging technology resources, and current trends and changing policies, without having to wait for a major curriculum revision?
- What opportunities exist for students in all programs to participate in collaborative interprofessional practice?
- To what extent are students exposed to the role of the nurse in nontraditional, as well as traditional, settings?
- What opportunities exist for students to take electives or to choose course assignments or activities that match their interests and individual learning goals?
- To what extent can faculty members, students, and alumni identify the features of the program that are truly innovative and serve to distinguish it from other programs?
- To what extent have faculty members used innovative approaches in the design and implementation of the course(s) for which they are responsible?
- In what ways is the curriculum regularly reviewed – with input from faculty members, students, and external stakeholders – and refined/revised as needed to incorporate current societal and healthcare trends and issues, research findings, innovative practices, and local as well as national and global perspectives?

The curriculum provides learning activities that enhance students' abilities to think critically, reflect thoughtfully, and provide culturally sensitive, evidence-based nursing care to diverse populations.

- What kinds of immersion-like learning experiences with individuals from cultures other than their own are designed for all students?
- What opportunities do students have to interact with patients/families, healthcare providers, faculty members, and peers who are diverse in terms of their culture, lifestyles, beliefs, and/or other characteristics?
- How do faculty members draw on learning experiences to enhance students' abilities to be culturally sensitive in the care they provide?
- To what extent do students consider and address social determinants of health when planning and providing care?
- How do faculty members help students heighten their awareness of their own values, unconscious biases, and stereotyping, particularly as they relate to inclusion, equity, and diversity?
- How are faculty members prepared to teach diverse student populations from a culturally sensitive, evidence-based perspective?
- To what extent does the curriculum align with the nursing program's and parent institution's vision, mission, and shared values of diversity, equity, inclusion, and civility?

The curriculum emphasizes students' values development, identity formation, caring for self, commitment to lifelong learning, critical thinking, ethical and evidence-based practice, and creativity.

- How much attention is paid throughout the curriculum to self-reflection, values clarification, analysis of what it means to be a nurse in the 21st century, and developing and living one's commitments to the profession, lifelong learning, career development, and similar or related factors?
- To what extent are students allowed and encouraged to be creative?
- How do faculty members respond to student diversity, students' unique approaches to doing assignments, and the individualized ways students learn, think, and set priorities?
- What learning activities are planned throughout the curriculum to help students develop role transition skills?
- In what ways do faculty members attend to and promote students' well-being?

The curriculum provides learning experiences that prepare graduates to assume roles that are essential to quality nursing practice, including but not limited to roles of care provider, advocate for those in need, teacher, communicator, change agent, care coordinator, member of intra- and interprofessional teams, user of information technology, collaborator, decision-maker, leader, and evolving scholar.

- What learning experiences give students the opportunity to develop competence and confidence in their ability to advocate for patients and families, teach individuals and groups about health care, serve as members and leaders of teams, facilitate change, manage conflict, and make decisions that affect their own well-being and the health of the patients and families for whom they care?
- What opportunities are provided to help students develop as leaders who can envision a preferred future and work collaboratively with others to facilitate change that makes the vision a reality?
- To what extent do students engage in scholarly activities – on their own, in collaboration with fellow students, or as part of faculty members' scholarly endeavors?
- How are students helped to develop confidence in their ability to use technological resources?
- How are students helped to find, judge, and use information, as well as manage large amounts of information?
- How do faculty members help students develop their writing skills, ability to speak to groups, ability to argue convincingly (or present a civil counter-argument), ability to listen effectively, ability to use social media effectively and appropriately, and other effective communication skills?
- To what extent do faculty members refer students to institutional resources (e.g., writing center, counseling center) as needed to support their development?

The curriculum provides learning experiences that support evidence-based practice, interprofessional approaches to care, student achievement of clinical competence, and, as appropriate, competence in a specialty role.

- To what extent do experiential (clinical, laboratory, and simulation) experiences help students develop their ability to provide culturally competent, evidence-based care to patients, families, and communities experiencing a wide range of health problems?
- What learning activities are designed to help graduate students develop competence in the full scope of their new role (e.g., advanced practitioner, educator, administrator, consultant, researcher), as members and leaders of intra- and interprofessional teams, and as professionals whose services (e.g., primary care, public health, teaching, curriculum development) are evidence based?

HALLMARKS AND INDICATORS RELATED TO INNOVATIVE, EVIDENCE-BASED APPROACHES TO FACILITATE AND EVALUATE LEARNING

Strategies used to facilitate and evaluate learning by a diverse student population are innovative and varied.

- To what extent are strategies to facilitate learning varied to meet the needs of diverse student populations?
- To what extent are strategies to facilitate learning aligned with student and program learning outcomes?
- In what ways are emerging trends in teaching and learning (e.g., online learning, self-directed study, technology, simulation) used by faculty members to facilitate and evaluate learning?
- In what ways do faculty members appraise evidence that supports their selection of strategies to facilitate and evaluate learning?

Faculty members engage in collegial dialogue and interact with students and colleagues in nursing and other professions to promote and develop strategies to facilitate and evaluate learning.

- In what ways are informal, open forum opportunities in place where faculty members, students, and clinical partners discuss and evaluate the effectiveness of current strategies to facilitate and evaluate learning?
- To what extent are student evaluations of teaching and peer review findings used to stimulate dialogue about the nature of excellence and innovation in nursing education?
- In what ways are regular discussions among faculty members about strategies to facilitate and evaluate learning incorporated into courses?

Strategies to facilitate and evaluate learning used by faculty members are evidence based.

- To what extent do faculty members use evidence from nursing and other disciplines to design strategies to facilitate and evaluate learning?
- To what extent do faculty members systematically document the effectiveness of strategies used to facilitate and evaluate learning in an effort to develop evidence that underlies teaching practices?

HALLMARKS AND INDICATORS RELATED TO RESOURCES TO SUPPORT PROGRAM GOAL ATTAINMENT

Partnerships in which the program is engaged promote excellence in nursing education, enhance the profession, benefit the community, enhance learning opportunities, and facilitate/support research/ scholarship initiatives.

- What are the criteria used to determine the agencies/organizations with which the nursing program will partner?
- How are partners engaged with faculty members and students to achieve excellence in the nursing program?

Technology is used effectively to facilitate, support, and evaluate student learning, faculty development, research/scholarship, and support services.

- How are faculty members and students prepared for/supported in the use of technology to facilitate and evaluate learning?
- What commitment has the nursing program made to integrate the use of technology throughout the program?
- To what extent is informatics integrated throughout the program to ensure that students are prepared for the current technology-driven practice world?

Student support services are culturally sensitive and empower students during the recruitment, retention, progression, graduation, and career planning processes.

- To what extent do students report that the recruitment and admission process was a welcoming one that acknowledged their unique needs?
- To what extent do students express comfort about seeking out and using the student services that are available to them?
- To what extent do students report satisfaction with the extent of support they receive throughout the program, at graduation, and in relation to entering a new career?

Financial resources are available to support initiatives that enhance faculty competence, student success, innovation, and scholarly endeavors.

- To what extent do financial resources support visionary, long-range planning and creative initiatives?
- To what extent do financial resources support faculty development and certification as a nurse educator?
- To what extent do financial resources support continuous quality improvement of the program?
- To what extent do resources available to faculty members, students, and administrators support efforts to be innovative, continually develop as members of the nursing profession and the academic community, and enact needed change?
- In what ways does the institution provide resources to support faculty scholarly endeavors such as grant writing, publications, and presentations at regional and national conferences?
- What administrative and financial support is available for faculty members to be innovative and evidence based in their approach to teaching and learning as well as in their approach to the design, implementation, and evaluation of the curriculum?
- How do faculty members' workloads support their efforts to create a preferred future for nursing education, nursing practice, or nursing research?

HALLMARKS AND INDICATORS RELATED TO A COMMITMENT TO PEDAGOGICAL SCHOLARSHIP

Faculty members and students contribute to the development of the science of nursing education through the critique, use, dissemination, and/or conduct of various forms of scholarly endeavors.

- To what extent do faculty members and students at all levels discuss research findings related to teaching and learning?
- In what ways do faculty members promote scholarly inquiry related to nursing education by students and colleagues?
- In what ways are faculty members and students involved in scholarly endeavors related to teaching and learning that contribute to the development of the art and science of nursing education?

Faculty members and students explore the influence of student learning experiences on the health of the individuals and populations they serve in various healthcare settings.

- What strategies are used to systematically document the extent to which student learning experiences affect healthcare outcomes for the populations they serve?
- To what extent do leaders in partner healthcare facilities report improved patient care outcomes or more effective nursing practices in areas where students have extended learning experiences?
- To what extent do student learning experiences influence nursing practice and/or healthcare policies?
- To what extent does the nursing program attend to improving the health of selected populations through teaching and learning activities as strategic plans and annual program goals are formulated?

HALLMARKS AND INDICATORS RELATED TO EFFECTIVE INSTITUTIONAL AND PROFESSIONAL LEADERSHIP

Faculty members, administrators, and students provide the leadership needed to ensure that the culture of the school promotes excellence and a healthy work environment characterized by collegial dialogue, innovation, change, creativity, values development, and ethical behavior.

- To what extent do faculty members, administrators, students, and clinical partners engage in collegial dialogue about what constitutes a positive teaching/learning environment and the roles of faculty members and students in creating such an environment?
- To what extent do faculty members, administrators, students, and clinical partners collaborate to create learning environments that empower a diverse student population, promote creativity and innovation, and prepare graduates for today's uncertain, constantly changing healthcare environment?
- To what extent is the environment in which faculty members, administrators, students, and staff work safe, civil, and collegial?

Faculty members, administrators, students, and alumni are respected as leaders in the parent institution, as well as in local, state, regional, national, and/or international communities.

- To what extent do faculty members and administrators hold influential positions on institutional committees, task forces, policy-making groups, or other similar bodies?
- To what extent do students hold influential positions on program or institutional committees, task forces, or other similar bodies?
- How many faculty members, administrators, and alumni are appointed to, invited to serve on, or elected to respected boards, institutes, or other similar bodies (e.g., Presidential Committee on Aging, National Academy of Sciences [formerly IOM], healthcare partner boards or committees)?
- How frequently do students bring resolutions to the National Student Nurses Association (NSNA) or proposals to the nursing program or institution that will influence change?

Faculty members, administrators, students, and alumni are prepared for and assume leadership roles that advance quality nursing care; promote positive change, innovation, and excellence; and enhance the impact of the nursing profession.

- To what extent do faculty members, administrators, or alumni serve on committees or boards of healthcare partner institutions or other groups/organizations that address quality and nursing care issues?
- What awards or honors do faculty members, administrators, students, or alumni receive in recognition of their contributions to the institution, profession, local community, or health care?
- To what extent do the curriculum and faculty development activities focus on the development of leadership knowledge and skills?
- To what extent do faculty members, administrators, and student leaders mentor and help develop future leaders?
- What elements of the program ensure faculty members, administrators, students, and alumni are prepared to and do shape a new reality for nursing and nursing education?
- To what extent do faculty members, administrators, students, and clinical partners engage in discussions about what kind of future they envision for nursing and nursing education?

Appendix C
Self-Assessment Checklist

The *Self-Assessment Checklist* reflects the National League for Nursing's *Hallmarks of Excellence in Nursing Education©*. The questions posed are indicators that faculty could use to determine the extent to which they are achieving each Hallmark and, thereby, achieving excellence in their nursing education program(s).

This checklist is envisioned to be used as a stimulus for serious reflection by faculty and nursing education administrators about the nature of schooling, teaching, and learning in their own environments. Such reflection and honest self-appraisal leads to proposals on how to transform the educational environment in the school such that excellence is attained.

ENGAGED STUDENTS		
Students are excited about learning and exhibit a spirit of inquiry as well as a commitment to lifelong learning.		
Indicator	Strengths	Needs Improvement
To what extent do students appraise evidence and use the information discovered to contribute to class and clinical discussions?		
In what ways do students brainstorm together about concepts such as those presented in class and introduced in various references and clinical experiences?		
To what extent do students question if current practices (e.g., approaches to patient care, the way communication occurs on clinical units, existing policies) are based on research and evidence?		
Do students ask "What if" questions?		
In what ways do students demonstrate enthusiasm about continued learning and professional development?		

ENGAGED STUDENTS

Students are committed to innovation, continuous quality/performance improvement, and excellence.

Indicator	Strengths	Needs Improvement
To what extent do students respond to critical/constructive feedback and then use that feedback to make improvements in their performance?		
In what ways are students open to trying new things?		
In what ways are students stimulated in their learning when innovative teaching strategies are integrated into the classroom, lab, and/or clinical setting?		
In what ways do students reflect on their own performance and experiences in order to be proactive in implementing improved performance?		
In what ways do students observe for areas of quality improvement within systems and suggest appropriate solutions?		
In what ways are students incorporating technology to make improvements in their performance?		

ENGAGED STUDENTS

Students are committed to the professional nursing role including advancement in leadership, scholarship, and mentoring.

Indicator	Strengths	Needs Improvement
In what ways do students express anticipatory excitement about professional identity formation, continuing their education, pursuing graduate study, assuming leadership roles in their employment settings and in the profession, serving as mentors, and becoming actively involved in professional associations? How do they express excitement about the contributions they hope to make to the nursing profession?		
In what ways do students propose a realistic short- and long-term career trajectory for themselves?		
To what extent do students collaborate with others to create environments that are civil, inclusive, respectful, and promote excellence?		
In what ways do students provide evidence of seeing themselves as being responsible for advancing the profession of nursing?		

DIVERSE, WELL-PREPARED FACULTY

The faculty complement is composed of diverse individuals who are leaders and/or have expertise in clinical practice, education, interprofessional collaboration, and research/scholarship consistent with the institution's mission and vision.

Indicator	Strengths	Needs Improvement
To what extent does the faculty complement reflect diversity, including but not limited to race, ethnicity, gender, and educational background?		
To what extent do hiring practices help to create a faculty complement that reflects expertise in education, clinical practice, interprofessional collaboration, and/or research/scholarship?		
To what extent do faculty members' job responsibility statements specifically address the expert behaviors required for the role of educator, clinician, and researcher/scholar?		

DIVERSE, WELL-PREPARED FACULTY

The unique contributions of each faculty member in teaching, service, research/scholarship, and practice that facilitate achievement of the program's mission and goals are valued, rewarded, and recognized.

Indicator	Strengths	Needs Improvement
To what are the unique contributions of faculty members with varied areas of expertise valued, rewarded, and recognized?		

- Expertise in education
- Expertise in clinical practice
- Expertise in research/scholarship
- Expertise in interprofessional collaboration
- Expertise in administration and/or management

DIVERSE, WELL-PREPARED FACULTY

Faculty members are accountable for promoting excellence, creating civil and inclusive environments, and providing leadership in their area(s) of expertise.

Indicator	Strengths	Needs Improvement
How are faculty members expected to demonstrate expertise and promote diversity?		
How do expert faculty members provide leadership and mentoring to other faculty members regarding their area(s) of expertise?		
In what ways are faculty members held accountable to fulfill expectations related to diversity, excellence, and providing leadership in their area(s) of expertise?		
In what ways do faculty members actively work to promote academic integrity and sustain an environment of civility and inclusivity?		
To what extent have faculty members made a commitment to challenge traditional approaches to nursing education and implement innovative, evidence-based approaches?		

DIVERSE, WELL-PREPARED FACULTY

Faculty members model a commitment to lifelong learning, involvement in professional and community organizations, and scholarly activities.

Indicator	Strengths	Needs Improvement
To what extent do faculty members demonstrate an openness to embracing and leading change in the learning environment and acquiring needed faculty competencies to create a preferred future in nursing?		
To what extent are faculty members expected to continue learning and acquiring knowledge in their area(s) of expertise through continuing education courses, certifications, post-master's courses, post-doctoral courses, or other formal or informal education?		
To what extent do faculty members make significant contributions to local, state, regional, national, and/or international professional organizations?		
To what extent do faculty members express excitement about a professional career in nursing when talking with students, with one another, and with others in and outside the profession?		

DIVERSE, WELL-PREPARED FACULTY

All faculty members have structured preparation for the faculty role, including competence in teaching, scholarship, and service.

Indicator	Strengths	Needs Improvement
Do all full-time, part-time, and adjunct faculty members receive an in-depth orientation to the faculty role?		
What forms of membership are provided to assist faculty members as they progress in their careers?		
Is an established set of faculty competencies used to prepare individuals for the faculty role and help them maintain competence or expertise in that role?		

A CULTURE OF CONTINUOUS QUALITY IMPROVEMENT

The program engages on a variety of activities that promote quality and excellence, including accreditation by national nursing accreditation bodies.

Indicator	Strengths	Needs Improvement
In what ways does the school's strategic plan reflect findings from the continuous quality improvement process in which faculty members, students, administrators, alumni, and community partners participate?		
To what extent does the program have a process to support faculty research/scholarship; attendance at local, national, and international conferences; and faculty development events?		
Does each program seek and maintain national nursing accreditation?		
To what extent are accreditation standards used to guide program evaluation and develop a culture of continuous quality improvement of the nursing program?		

A CULTURE OF CONTINUOUS QUALITY IMPROVEMENT

Program design, implementation, and evaluation are continuously reviewed and revised to achieve and maintain excellence.

Indicator	Strengths	Needs Improvement
Is there a mechanism in place for continuous review of program design, implementation, and evaluation?		
In what ways are curricular revisions made that allow the program to keep current with changes and trends in health care, healthcare economics, healthcare delivery systems, education, national standards and competencies, societal norms, and expectations of nurses?		
In what ways are faculty members, along with administrators, engaged in discussion about quality improvement as part of their role within the organization?		
To what extent are program revisions based on findings from the continuous review of program design, implementation, and evaluation?		
To what extent do faculty members and students systematically evaluate the impact of innovative teaching strategies and curriculum approaches on (1) student learning outcomes, student satisfaction, and other student-centered outcomes; and (2) faculty satisfaction, scholarship, and professional growth?		

INNOVATIVE, EVIDENCE-BASED CURRICULUM

The curriculum is designed to help students achieve stated program outcomes, reflects current societal and healthcare trends and issues, and is responsive to change and evolving societal needs. The curriculum also embeds evidence-based information, reflects research findings and innovative practices, attends to the evolving role of the nurse in a variety of settings, is flexible and innovative, and incorporates local, national, and global perspectives.

Indicator	Strengths	Needs Improvement
What opportunities are available for students to take courses in a sequence that makes sense to them or allows them to pursue study in areas in which they have learning needs?		
To what extent is the curriculum offered in flexible formats (e.g., part-time/full-time, day/evening, on-line/face-to face/hybrid) to meet the individualized needs of the students?		
To what extent is the curriculum flexible, allow-ing faculty members to address new issues, new knowledge and scientific developments, emerg-ing technology resources, and current trends and changing policies, without having to wait for a major curriculum revision?		
What opportunities exist for students in all programs to participate in collaborative interprofessional practice?		
To what extent are students exposed to the role of the nurse in nontraditional, as well as traditional, settings?		
What opportunities exist for students to take electives or to choose course assignments or activities that match their interests and individual learning goals?		
To what extent can faculty members, students, and alumni identify the features of the program that are truly innovative and serve to distinguish it from other programs?		
To what extent have faculty members used innova-tive approaches in the design and implementation of the course(s) for which they are responsible?		
In what ways is the curriculum regularly reviewed – with input from faculty members, students, and ex-ternal stakeholders – and refined/revised as needed to incorporate current societal and healthcare trends and issues, research findings, innovative practices, and local as well as national and global perspectives?		

INNOVATIVE, EVIDENCE-BASED CURRICULUM

The curriculum provides learning activities that enhance students' abilities to think critically, reflect thoughtfully, and provide culturally sensitive, evidence-based nursing care to diverse populations.

Indicator	Strengths	Needs Improvement
What kinds of immersion-like learning experiences with individuals from cultures other than their own are designed for all students?		
What opportunities do students have to interact with patients/families, healthcare providers, or faculty members and peers who are diverse in terms of their culture, lifestyles, beliefs, and/or other characteristics?		
How do faculty members draw on learning experiences to enhance students' abilities to be culturally sensitive in the care they provide?		
To what extent do students consider and address social determinants of health when planning and providing care?		
How do faculty members help students heighten their awareness of their own values, unconscious biases, and stereotyping, particularly as they relate to inclusion, equity, and diversity?		
How are faculty members prepared to teach diverse student populations from a culturally sensitive, evidence-based perspective?		
To what extent does the curriculum align with the nursing program's and parent institution's vision, mission, and shared values of diversity, equity, inclusion, and civility?		

INNOVATIVE, EVIDENCE-BASED CURRICULUM

The curriculum emphasizes students' values development, identity formation, caring for self, commitment to lifelong learning, critical thinking, ethical and evidence-based practice, and creativity.

Indicator	Strengths	Needs Improvement
How much attention is paid throughout the curriculum to self-reflection, values clarification, analysis of what it means to be a nurse in the 21st century, and developing and living one's commitments to the profession, lifelong learning, career development, and similar or related factors?		
To what extent are students allowed and encouraged to be creative?		
How do faculty members respond to student diversity, students' unique approaches to doing assignments, and the individualized ways students learn, think, and set priorities?		
What learning activities are planned throughout the curriculum to help students develop role transition skills?		
In what ways do faculty members attend to and promote students' well-being?		

INNOVATIVE, EVIDENCE-BASED CURRICULUM

The curriculum provides learning experiences that prepare graduates to assume roles that are essential to quality nursing practice, including but not limited to roles of care provider, advocate for those in need, teacher, communicator, change agent, care coordinator, member of intra- and interprofessional teams, user of information technology, collaborator, decision-maker, leader, and evolving scholar.

Indicator	Strengths	Needs Improvement
What learning experience gives students the opportunity to develop competence and confidence in their ability to advocate for patients and families, teach individuals and groups about health care, serve as members and leaders of teams, facilitate change, manage conflict, and make decisions that affect their own well-being and the health of the patients and families for whom they care?		
What opportunities are provided to help students develop as leaders who can envision a preferred future and work collaboratively with others to facilitate change that makes the vision a reality?		
To what extent do students engage in scholarly activities on their own, in collaboration with fellow students, or as part of the faculty members' scholarly endeavors?		
How are students helped to develop confidence in their ability to use technological resources?		
How are students helped to find, judge, and use information, as well as manage large amounts of information?		
How do faculty members help students develop their writing skills, ability to speak to groups, ability to argue convincingly (or present a civil counter-argument), ability to listen effectively, ability to use social media effectively and appropriately, and other effective communication skills?		
To what extent do faculty members refer students to institutional resources (e.g., writing center, counseling center) as needed to support their development?		

INNOVATIVE, EVIDENCE-BASED CURRICULUM

The curriculum provides learning experiences that support evidence-based practice, interprofessional approaches to care, student achievement of clinical competence, and, as appropriate, competence in a specialty role.

Indicator	Strengths	Needs Improvement
To what extent do experiential (clinical, laboratory, and simulation) experiences help students develop their ability to provide culturally competent, evidence-based care to patients, families, and communities experiencing a wide range of health problems?		
What learning activities are designed to help graduate students develop competence in the full scope of their new role (e.g., advanced practitioner, educator, administrator, consultant, researcher), as members and leaders of intra- and interprofessional teams, and as professionals whose services (e.g., primary care, public health, teaching, curriculum development) are evidence based?		

INNOVATIVE, EVIDENCE-BASED APPROACHES TO FACILITATE AND EVALUATE LEARNING

Strategies used to facilitate and evaluate learning by a diverse student population are innovative and varied.

Indicator	Strengths	Needs Improvement
To what extent are strategies to facilitate learning varied to meet the needs of diverse student populations?		
To what extent are strategies to facilitate learning aligned with student and program learning outcomes?		
In what ways are emerging trends in teaching and learning (e.g., online learning, self-directed study, technology, simulation) used by faculty members to facilitate and evaluate learning?		
In what ways do faculty members appraise evidence that supports their selection of strategies to facilitate and evaluate learning?		

INNOVATIVE, EVIDENCE-BASED APPROACHES TO FACILITATE AND EVALUATE LEARNING

Faculty members engage in collegial dialogue and interact with students and colleagues in nursing and other professions to promote and develop strategies to facilitate and evaluate learning.

Indicator	Strengths	Needs Improvement
In what ways are informal, open forum opportunities in place where faculty members, students, and clinical partners discuss and evaluate the effectiveness of current strategies to facilitate and evaluate learning?		
To what extent are student evaluations of teaching and peer review findings used to stimulate dialogue about the nature of excellence and innovation in nursing education?		
In what ways are regular discussions among faculty members about strategies to facilitate and evaluate learning incorporated into courses?		

INNOVATIVE, EVIDENCE-BASED APPROACHES TO FACILITATE AND EVALUATE LEARNING

Strategies to facilitate and evaluate learning used by faculty members are evidence based.

Indicator	Strengths	Needs Improvement
To what extent do faculty members use evidence from nursing and other disciplines to design strategies to facilitate and evaluate learning?		
To what extent do faculty members systematically document the effectiveness of strategies used to facilitate and evaluate learning in an effort to develop evidence that underlies teaching practices?		

RESOURCES TO SUPPORT PROGRAM GOAL ATTAINMENT

Partnerships in which the program is engaged promote excellence in nursing education, enhance the profession, benefit the community, enhance learning opportunities, and facilitate/support research/ scholarship initiatives.

Indicator	Strengths	Needs Improvement
What are the criteria used to determine the agencies/organizations with which the nursing program will partner?		
How are partners engaged with faculty members and students to achieve excellence in the nursing program?		

RESOURCES TO SUPPORT PROGRAM GOAL ATTAINMENT

Technology is used effectively to facilitate, support, and evaluate student learning, faculty development, research/scholarship, and support services.

Indicator	Strengths	Needs Improvement
How are faculty members and students prepared for/supported in the use of technology to facilitate and evaluate learning?		
What commitment has the nursing program made to integrate the use of technology throughout the program?		
To what extent is informatics integrated throughout the program to ensure that students are prepared for the current technology-driven world?		

RESOURCES TO SUPPORT PROGRAM GOAL ATTAINMENT

Student support services are culturally sensitive and empower students during the recruitment, retention, progression, graduation, and career planning process.

Indicator	Strengths	Needs Improvement
To what extent do students report that the recruitment and admission process was a welcoming one that acknowledged their unique needs?		
To what extent do students express comfort about seeking out and using the student services that are available to them?		
To what extent do students report satisfaction with the extent of support they receive throughout the program, at graduation, and in relation to entering a new career?		

RESOURCES TO SUPPORT PROGRAM GOAL ATTAINMENT

Financial resources are available to support initiatives that enhance faculty competence, student success, innovation, and scholarly endeavors.

Indicator	Strengths	Needs Improvement
To what extent do financial resources support visionary, long-range planning and creative initiatives?		
To what extent do financial resources support faculty development and certification as a nurse educator?		
To what extent do financial resources support continuous quality improvement of the program?		
To what extent do resources available to faculty members, students, and administrators support efforts to be innovative, continually develop as members of the nursing profession and the academic community, and enact needed change?		
In what ways does the institution provide resources to support faculty scholarly endeavors such as grant writing, publications, and presentations at regional and national conferences?		
What administrative and financial support is available for faculty members to be innovative and evidence based in their approach to teaching and learning as well as in their approach to the design, implementation, and evaluation of the curriculum?		
How do faculty members' workloads support their efforts to create a preferred future for nursing education, nursing practice, or nursing research?		

COMMITMENT TO PEDAGOGICAL SCHOLARSHIP

Faculty members and students contribute to the development of the science of nursing education through the critique, use, dissemination, and/or conduct of various forms of scholarly endeavors.

Indicator	Strengths	Needs Improvement
To what extent do faculty members and students at all levels discuss research findings related to teaching and learning?		
In what ways do faculty members promote scholarly inquiry related to nursing education by students and colleagues?		
In what ways are faculty members and students involved in scholarly endeavors related to teaching and learning that contribute to the development of the art and science of nursing education?		

COMMITMENT TO PEDAGOGICAL SCHOLARSHIP

Faculty members and students explore the influence of student learning experiences on the health of the individuals and populations they serve in various healthcare settings.

Indicator	Strengths	Needs Improvement
What strategies are used to systematically document the extent to which student learning experiences affect healthcare outcomes for the populations they serve?		
To what extent do leaders in partner healthcare facilities report improved patient care outcomes or more effective nursing practices in areas where students have extended learning experiences?		
To what extent do student learning experiences influence nursing practice and/or healthcare policies?		
To what extent does the nursing program attend to improving the health of selected populations through teaching and learning activities as strategic plans and annual program goals are formulated?		

EFFECTIVE INSTITUTIONAL AND PROFESSIONAL LEADERSHIP

Faculty members, administrators, and students provide the leadership needed to ensure that the culture of the school promotes excellence and a healthy work environment characterized by collegial dialogue, innovation, change, creativity, values development, and ethical behavior.

Indicator	Strengths	Needs Improvement
To what extent do faculty members, administrators, students, and clinical partners engage in collegial dialogue about what constitutes a positive teaching/ learning environment and the roles of faculty members and students in creating such an environment?		
To what extent do faculty members, administrators, students, and clinical partners collaborate to create learning environments that empower a diverse student population, promote creativity and innovation, and prepare graduates for today's uncertain, constantly changing healthcare environment?		
To what extent is the environment in which faculty members, administrators, students, and staff work safe, civil, and collegial?		

EFFECTIVE INSTITUTIONAL
AND PROFESSIONAL LEADERSHIP

Faculty members, administrators, students, and alumni are respected as leaders in the parent institution, as well as in local, state, regional, national, and/or international communities.

Indicator	Strengths	Needs Improvement
To what extent do faculty members and administrators hold influential positions on institutional committees, task forces, policy-making groups, or other similar bodies?		
To what extent do students hold influential positions on program or institutional committees, task forces, or other similar bodies?		
How many faculty members, administrators, and alumni are appointed to, invited to serve on, or elected to respected boards, institutes, or other similar bodies (e.g., Presidential Committee on Aging, National Academy of Sciences [formerly IOM], healthcare partner boards or committees)?		
How frequently do students bring resolutions to the National Student Nurses Association (NSNA) or proposals to the nursing program or institution that will influence change?		

EFFECTIVE INSTITUTIONAL AND PROFESSIONAL LEADERSHIP

Faculty members, administrators, students, and alumni are prepared for and assume leadership roles that advance quality nursing care; promote positive change, innovation, and excellence; and enhance the impact of the nursing profession.

Indicator	Strengths	Needs Improvement
To what extent do faculty members, administrators, or alumni serve in committees or boards of health-care partner institutions or other groups/organizations that address quality nursing care issues?		
What awards or honors do faculty members, administrators, students, or alumni receive in recognition of their contributions to the institution, profession, local community, or health care?		
To what extent do the curriculum and faculty development activities focus on the development of leadership knowledge and skills?		
To what extent do faculty members, administrators, and student leaders mentor and help develop future leaders?		
What elements of the program ensure faculty members, administrators, students, and alumni are prepared to and do shape a new reality for nursing and nursing education?		
To what extent do faculty members, administrators, students, and clinical partners engage in discussions about what kind of future they envision for nursing and nursing education?		

Glossary

Civility An "authentic respect for others when expressing disagreement, disparity, or controversy" (Clark & Carnosso, 2008, p. 13). Attributes include being fully present, respecting one another, honoring differences, and engaging in genuine discourse with a sincere intention to seek common ground (Clark & Carnosso, 2008).

Competence The application of knowledge and interpersonal, decision-making, and psychomotor skills in the performance of a task or implementation of a role.

Continuous Quality/Performance Improvement A comprehensive, sustained, and integrative approach to assessment and evaluation that aims toward continual improvement and renewal of an individual and/or a total system.

Creativity A process that calls upon an individual's curiosity, inquisitiveness, and ability to generate new ideas and perspectives that result in products and practices that are unique but also useful.

Curriculum The interaction among learners, teachers, and knowledge – occurring in an academic environment – that is designed to accomplish goals identified by the learners, the teachers, and the profession the learners expect to enter. It is more than a collection of courses or the sequencing of learning experiences, and it is more than an outline of the content to be "covered" during an academic program.

Enhancing Cultural Sensitivity Purposefully designed learning experiences that help students gain greater understanding of, insight to, and sensitivity regarding (1) the practices and beliefs of people whose culture, history, and life experiences are different from their own, and (2) the meaning that people give to their life experiences.

Ethical Behavior A system of moral conduct based on one's personal beliefs, values, customs, and character, as well as those of one 's profession.

Evidence-based Nursing Care/Practice The provision of nursing care to individuals, groups, and communities that evolves from the systematic integration of research findings related to a particular clinical problem. Intervention strategies are designed based on the evidence garnered through research, questions are raised about clinical practices that lead to new research endeavors, and the effectiveness of interventions are systematically evaluated in an effort to continually improve care.

Evidence-based Teaching Practice Using systematically developed and appropriately integrated research as the foundation for curriculum design, selection of strategies to facilitate and evaluate learning, advisement practices, and other elements of the educational enterprise.

Excellence "Striving to be the very best you can be in everything you do – not because some . . . 'authority figure' [demands it], but because you can't imagine functioning in any other way. It means setting high standards for yourself and the groups in which you are involved, holding yourself to those standards despite challenges or pressures to reduce or lower them, and not being satisfied with anything less than the very best" (Grossman & Valiga, 2021, p. 255).

Expertise Having or displaying special skill, knowledge, or mastery of a particular subject, derived from extensive training or experience.

Global Perspective Knowledge about and critical understanding of global issues that enable an individual to (1) effectively address those issues; (2) acquire values that give priority to ecological sustainability, global interdependence, social justice for all the world's people, peace, human rights, and mutually beneficial processes of economic, social, and cultural development; (3) develop the will and ability to act as mature, responsible citizens of the world; and (4) develop a commitment to creating acceptable futures for themselves, their communities, and the world. Such a perspective is critical in light of the increasing connectivity and interdependence of the world's social, economic, educational, and other systems.

Informatics In nursing, the integration of "nursing science with multiple information and analytical sciences to identify, define, manage and communicate data, information, knowledge and wisdom in nursing practice" (Healthcare Information and Management Systems Society, 2019).

Innovation/Innovative Practices The spark of insight that leads an individual to investigate an issue or phenomenon and that is usually shaped by an observation of what appears to be true or the creative jolt of a new idea. Innovation is driven by a commitment to excellence and continuous improvement, and it is based on curiosity, the willingness to take risks, experimenting to test assumptions, questioning and challenging the status quo, and recognizing and taking advantage of opportunity.

Interprofessional Education (IPE) Partnerships where health profession educators and healthcare providers "break down the traditional silo-approach to health professions education and practice" and, instead, learn with, from, and about each other in order to "work together to meet the demands of transforming processes of care delivery and the challenges in educating and training the next generation of health professionals" (National Center for Interprofessional Education, n.d., p. 1).

Leadership A complex, multifaceted phenomenon that involves the elements of "vision, communication skills, trust, change, courage, stewardship, and developing and renewing followers" (Grossman & Valiga, 2021, p. 27). Tasks assumed by the individual who chooses or agrees to "make a difference in the lives of others and in the directions of groups and organizations" (Grossman & Valiga, 2017, p. 28) include envisioning goals, affirming values, motivating, managing, achieving a workable unity, explaining, serving as a symbol, representing the group, and renewing (Gardner, 1990).

Lifelong Learning The provision or use of both formal and informal learning opportunities throughout one's life to foster continuous development, enhancement of the knowledge and skills needed to implement one's professional role, and personal fulfillment.

Partner/Partnerships An alliance between individuals or groups in which all parties mutually develop goals, collaborate to achieve those goals, and benefit from the alliance.

Pedagogical Scholarship Systematic inquiry into all aspects of the teaching/learning process, including how students learn, effective strategies to facilitate and evaluate learning, curriculum design and implementation, program outcomes, learner outcomes, environments that enhance learning, and other components of the educational enterprise.

Preferred Future for Nursing "What should happen or what we would like to see evolve . . . Creat[ing] the future we want and orchestrat[ing] events and situations to achieve the goals we set for ourselves and to fulfill the roles we envision for ourselves" (Valiga, 1994, p. 86).

Reward Recompense made to or received by an individual for some service or merit. In the educational environment, traditional faculty rewards are tenure, promotion, and salary increase. Other types of rewards for faculty are those that derive from factors that motivate individuals to pursue the faculty role, including autonomy, belonging to a community of scholars, recognition, and efficacy (i.e., having an impact on one's environment).

Science of Nursing Education An integrated, systematically developed body of knowledge that "address[es] questions related to student learning, new pedagogies, graduate competencies, program outcomes, innovative clinical teaching models, effective student advisement strategies, recruitment and retention strategies, and other elements of quality nursing education" (Tanner, 2003, p. 3).

Spirit of Inquiry "A persistent sense of curiosity that informs both learning and practice. [Those] infused by a spirit of inquiry will raise questions, challenge traditional and existing practices, seek creative approaches to problem[-solving]." It "engenders innovative thinking and extends possibilities for discovering novel solutions in both ambiguous, uncertain, and unpredictable situations [and] suggests to some degree, a childlike sense of wonder" (National League for Nursing, 2010, p. 36).

Structured Preparation for the Faculty Role "Nursing education is a specialized area of practice, and nurse educators who understand and implement discipline-specific pedagogy are the vital link to a future workforce that will lead health care reform . . . it is critical that graduate programs in nursing, including master's and research and practice doctorates, prepare graduates with the knowledge, attitudes, and skills to teach, to provide leadership for transforming education and health care systems, and to conduct and translate research on salient nursing education phenomena. Achieving this goal is critical to justify the public's trust in our profession. In addition, the profession has the obligation to prepare nurse educators who can facilitate the learning of the next generation of nurses to ensure safe, quality care to changing populations in a variety of health care settings" (Patterson, 2017, p. 366).

Student Support Services Services that promote the comprehensive development of the student and help strengthen learning outcomes by reinforcing and extending the educational institution's influence beyond the classroom. Such services include but are not limited to admissions, financial aid, registration, orientation, advisement, tutoring, counseling, discipline, health, housing, placement, student organizations and activities, cultural programming, childcare, security, and athletics.

Technology The use of science and the application of scientific principles to any situation, often involving the use of sophisticated equipment and computers.

Traditional Approaches to Nursing Education Teacher-directed, highly structured approaches that rely heavily on the delivery of content through lecture, the evaluation of learning through multiple-choice examinations, highly structured and relatively inflexible curriculum designs, and strict adherence to policies. The focus is on cognitive gain, "covering" content, a simple-to-complex approach, problem-solving, and efficiency.

Values Development The evolution of personal principles, character, and customs that provide the framework for making decisions about one's daily actions. Values are the product of one's life experiences, give meaning and direction to life, and are influenced by family, friends, religion, culture, environment, education, and other factors.

References

Clark, C. M., & Carnosso, S. (2008). Civility: A concept analysis. *The Journal of Theory Construction & Testing, 12*(1), 11–15.

Gardner, J. W. (1990). *On leadership*. Simon & Schuster.

Grossman, S. C., & Valiga, T. M. (2017). *The new leadership challenge: Creating the future of nursing* (5th ed.). F.A. Davis.

Grossman, S. C., & Valiga, T. M. (2021). *The new leadership challenge: Creating the future of nursing* (6th ed.). F.A. Davis.

Healthcare Information and Management Systems Society. (2019). What is nursing informatics? https://www.himss.org/resources/what-nursing-informatics

National Center for Interprofessional Practice and Education. (n.d.). Introduction. https://macyfoundation.org/stories/national-center-for-interprofessional-practice-and-education

National League for Nursing. (2010). *Outcomes and competencies for graduates of practical/vocational, diploma, associate degree, baccalaureate, master's, practice doctorate, and research doctorate programs in nursing.* Author.

Patterson, B. (2017). NLN releases a vision for graduate preparation for academic nurse educators. *Nursing Education Perspectives, 38*(6), 366. https://doi.org/10.1097/01.NEP.0000000000000242

Tanner, C. A. (2003). Science and nursing education [Editorial]. *Journal of Nursing Education, 42*(1), 3–4.

Valiga, T. M. (1994). Leadership for the future. *Holistic Nursing Practice, 9*(1), 83–90. http://doi.org/10.1097/00004650-199410000-00013